Praise for *This Is What You're Really Hungry For*

"We must examine how society's pressure for perfection affects our relationship to our bodies and how we use our time. Shapira's method is not another how-to fad, it is a system that brings us back to what is truly important—what it means to be physically and mentally healthy."

—Eve Rodsky, *New York Times* bestselling author of *Fair Play* and *Find Your Unicorn Space*

"*This Is What You're Really Hungry For* is for anyone wanting to get to the root of why you crave certain foods and how to develop new and lasting habits that are sustainable through a series of easy-to-follow rules that are guaranteed to kick-start your wellness journey like never before. Kim speaks to you as if she is a caring friend who truly wants the best for you and in a world full of harsh critiques, the toughest ones being ourselves! She lays out the 'whys'—why your gut is acting up, why you need to be aware of your food sensitivities, why mindfulness and a healthy relationship with food go hand in hand, and so much more. You deserve to take back your power when it comes to nutrition . . . So, drop the excuses and read this book!"

—Debbie Gibson, singer-songwriter and actress

"When you need something done, go to a busy person. Kim Shapira exhibits her boundless energy and insightfulness in her new book. This treatise is a unique approach to integrating the science and psychology of eating. Kim's words are straight from the heart. Her intent noble. A must read!"

—Bruce H. Zietz, MD, oncologist and hematology specialist

"Kim Shapira takes her clients on a journey of finding peace with food. Her method puts in place a fail-safe so we can learn to eat *only* what we love without it leading to weight gain. With her six simple rules, we can achieve whatever our body goals may be. Kim even goes so far as to share what will happen when we follow some—rather than all—of the rules. Kim Shapira's finest quality, though, is compassion and understanding for how complicated this food journey is for so many, and she guides with both kindness and expertise."

—Jenny Hutt, host of the *Just Jenny* podcast

"I have been in private internal medicine practice for 23 years and have had the privilege of working with Kim Shapira to improve the health of my patients. Her approach is not an elimination diet but more a life plan that reframes the relationship the patient has with eating. She introduced non-diet eating and recognition of the psychological connections with food prior to her predecessors. Her treatment plans work and are sustained. Kim has successfully helped many of my patients and her methods are not restrictive but more supportive."

—Monica Sarang, MD, internal medical physician

"Kim Shapira shares her fabulous approach to redefining body positivity and a healthy relationship with food. Her method and mentality about food and body changed a lot of my thinking. She helped me in so many ways."

—**Brittany Snow, actor, director, and founder of September Letters**

"Kim's very simple yet effective method has helped me maintain a healthy relationship with food for over ten years. After three pregnancies and many pounds to lose thereafter, I can confidently say that Kim's tips and tricks are an extremely effective way to see results as well as calm your mind when it comes to health."

—**Marla Sokoloff, actor, director, and mom of three girls**

"Kim Shapira is a gift! After many years of failed diets, cleanses, and one attempt to freeze the fat, I met Kim and she saved me—from myself. Her six simple rules completely changed my unhealthy relationship with my body and food. I've never been healthier or in better shape and I get to eat pizza! She's brilliant. This book is everything. You get to have pizza!"

—**Liz Astrof, award-winning executive producer and sitcom writer, creator of *Pivoting*, and author of *Stay-at-Work Mom***

"Kim's genius is her ability to inspire the adoption of transformative habits in those who have previously resorted to punishing and judging themselves and their relationship with food. Kim's book is the warm hug you need to kickstart your journey to self-love, and ultimately give up the fight with food. She step-by-step shows readers how to embrace food as the fuel our bodies need to reach new heights and live epic lives."

—**Elizabeth Pearson, nationally recognized executive coach to women in male-dominated fields and author of *Career Confinement***

"I applaud Kim Shapira for looking at our everyday diets, and how and why we eat, through an entirely new lens. As a clinical child psychologist, I highly recommend this six-step strategy to parents wanting to shape their children's health and food behaviors in a positive, self-affirming direction, free from peer pressure and societal dos and don'ts. It's a must-read for anyone raising a family at a time when childhood obesity and teen eating disorders are increasing at an alarming rate."

—**Dr. Myah Gittelson, PsyD, clinical psychologist**

"Kim Shapira's book is truly revolutionary . . . No need for confusing and contradictory diets. No need for fasting or following unhealthy food recommendations. Just use common sense and the easy steps described in Kim's digestible and enjoyable book."

—**Antoine Hage, MD, professor of medicine and cardiology at UCLA's David Geffin School of Medicine and Cedars-Sinai Smidt Heart Institute**

"Kim's approach to food and eating is fresh and modern. Her focus on creating positive habits versus counting calories or following a restrictive diet is something that appeals to me as a doctor. Getting people to understand why their approach and relationship with food is stressed is Kim's specialty and she does a brilliant job of breaking down tricky topics. *This is What You're Really Hungry For* is an actionable guide that will inspire adults and teens to adopt a healthier mindset around food and eating."

—Dr. Thaïs Aliabadi, physician, surgeon, and founder of Trimly

"I couldn't put Kim's book down and I've already worked with her as an in-person client. Kim is more like a nutritionist combined with a life coach. She won't let you beat yourself up . . . and believe me, I've tried! It doesn't feel like you're being restricted like so many other 'diets' and meal plans. She gives you all of the tools to know that you get a chance to reset with every meal . . . with every thought! If she was able to help *me* break my nightly 'I'm walking the dog at 11:00pm with a big pocketful of chocolate chips' habit, she can help *anyone*!"

—Larry Sullivan, actor

"As a fitness professional for over 15 years, it's unusual to read any truly ground-breaking approaches to eating. *This Is What You're Really Hungry For* does that starting on page one and keeps challenging everything we've been taught to believe about 'diet.' I wish everyone would throw out their scale and read this instead!"

—Amy Jordan, founder and CEO of WundaBar Pilates and WundaCore

"For years, Kim has approached her clients with her singular mix of common sense and compassion, wisdom and empathy, actionable rules that feel within reach, and progress that's both real and not too extreme. It's why she is the only voice that ever really breaks through all of the noise for me, the only expert I'd ever really trust. *This Is What You're Really Hungry For* is the peak of all that. Her guidance is a gift, rooted in her experience and given with a deep understanding of how people actually think about food and what it takes to make real change."

—Emily Jane Fox, national correspondent at *Vanity Fair* and cohost of *Inside the Hive*

"Kim Shapira has been working with my patients for years and is one of my most trusted referral resources. Her compassionate, evidence-based, real-life approach to supporting nutritional needs in a culture that confuses us is just unmatched. I'm so excited for this book and sharing these steps to true self love more widely."

—Suzanne Gilberg-Lenz, MD, board-certified in OB-GYN and integrative and holistic medicine

"Kim's careful guidance but strong vision for what it means to truly live a fulfilling and healthy life is the reason I am finally able to do so. Her book is thoughtful, inspiring, and an effortless read with an incredibly modern point of view. The rules are easy to follow and yet challenge us in the best of ways to want to do better and be better. I'm forever grateful that I found Kim Shapira and even more grateful that I can now carry her book with me through life."

—Bradley Bredeweg, creator of TV shows *The Fosters* and *Good Trouble*

This Is What You're Really Hungry For

This Is What You're Really Hungry For

Six Simple Rules to Transform Your Relationship with Food to Become Your Healthiest Self

KIM SHAPIRA

BenBella Books, Inc.
Dallas, TX

BENBELLA

BenBella Books, Inc.
10440 N. Central Expressway
Suite 800
Dallas, TX 75231
benbellabooks.com
Send feedback to feedback@benbellabooks.com

BenBella is a federally registered trademark.

Printed in the United States of America
10 9 8 7 6 5 4 3 2 1

Library of Congress Control Number: 2022060008
ISBN 9781637743416 (trade paperback)
ISBN 9781637743423 (electronic)

Editing by Alyn Wallace
Copyediting by Elizabeth Degenhard
Proofreading by Jenny Rosen and Sarah Vostok
Text design and composition by PerfecType, Nashville, TN
Cover design by Brigid Pearson
Cover image © Shutterstock / grey_and
Printed by Lake Book Manufacturing

To Matt:

*Thank you for giving me the courage to grow, for being my
biggest fan, and for believing in me before I did.*

To Olivia, Sophia, and Natasha:

*Thank you for letting me have the time and space to write this book. This book is
dedicated to the three of you, as you are, and always will be, my greatest teachers.*

To Mom and Dad:

*Thank you for teaching me to stand when I wanted to sit,
for your love and support, and for being mine.*

CONTENTS

RULE #4: TAKE 10,000 STEPS EVERY DAY

RULE #5: DRINK EIGHT CUPS OF WATER A DAY

RULE #6: GET SEVEN HOURS OF SLEEP

PUTTING IT ALL TOGETHER

FOREWORD BY KALEY CUOCO

Lemme start by saying, I am not a writer . . . like, at all! But when Kim asked me to write her foreword, I said yes because I know what it's like to struggle with weight, overeating, undereating, stress eating, and everything in between.

I have been in the public eye basically since I was sixteen years old, which is right when I met Kim. I was working on a little show called *8 Simple Rules* with John Ritter. I had worked a ton as a kid, but this was my first "big break," if you will. I didn't know what to do. I didn't know how to act, eat, work out, be an actor, or even be myself. It was all very new for me, and I truly needed some guidance.

It was strange because I was a young teen, now in a very adult job, surrounded by adults, and living a very adult life. I felt a bit lost. I was introduced to Kim by a publicist I had at the time. It was the best gift that the publicist ever gave to me. Kim helped me prioritize my health and start eating and thinking in a super positive way.

She has truly seen me through it all—all the ups and downs of life and what focusing on yourself can do to your mental health and your physical well-being. I have always considered her part therapist and part dietitian. While Kim and I would discuss food and when to eat based on my needs during the day, she was also very much helping me manage stress. Kim has always focused on my whole self, making sure I was taking deep breaths, moving my body, drinking my water, and helping with sleep, especially when I worked nights. Over the years, I have gone in and out of working with her, like a checkup, but whenever I truly need to get my body and brain back into gear, she is always the one I call.

Her method and outlook on food have always stayed the same: she made it easy to be anywhere in the world, free from worrying about what I was going to eat, and where I was going to eat it. Her outlook has truly never changed because it works—her focus has always been the same, to keep me balanced and healthy. Kim has been able to pinpoint what foods work for my body and what foods do not. No matter what, she always comes back to her six main rules. She knows what she is doing, and she keeps it simple. I remember when we first met and I was so nervous about what to eat, how much to eat, when to eat, blah, blah, blah. And she said to me, "Eat when you're hungry."

I thought, *Wow, that's it?* It seemed too simple, but that is because it was and still is.

I will never forget the first time Kim told me, way back when: "Eat half of your plate, take a breath, and if you are still hungry fifteen minutes later, eat more—that way, you'll know if you're actually hungry." (She also told me this about a month ago. Ha—because it still works to this day!) I tended to eat very quickly in a super distracted environment. I didn't even realize what was happening, but as a result, I would eat more than I needed and feel very full and sick, basically hurting myself. But because of her advice and guidance, I no longer do that.

All the things Kim taught me way back when I first started seeing her at sixteen years old are still things she teaches me and everyone else today. If it ain't broke, don't fix it.

Kim has helped me, and countless others, understand how to live a healthy, happy, consistent, satisfying life, and I promise with this book, she will help you, too.

NOT ANOTHER DIET BOOK: WHY USE THE KIM SHAPIRA METHOD?

You weren't allowed to leave the table before you cleaned your plate of Grandma's "tuna" casserole. Uncle Pete called you "chubby cheeks" at your high school graduation, so you skipped eating the cake with your face printed on it. You got ice cream every time you finished a dreaded piano lesson.

Our relationship with food starts as soon as we can chew it. It shows up in our earliest childhood memories as a confidant, a bully, a lover, and everything in between. With decades of emotionally charged history, is it any wonder that we forget that the true purpose of food is simply to fuel us? Identifying *why* we're eating is the key to losing weight and keeping it off; using food purposefully matters.

Now, you might be asking yourself, "How do *you* know what matters?" or maybe, "Who the heck are you to even tell me this?"

Hi. I'm Kim, and in the summer of 1986, I was a shy middle schooler whose life turned upside down because I got sick. I spent the next five years in and out of doctors' offices. It was scary and stressful, but when I look back, what I remember most is my intense appreciation for my team of doctors, nurses, family, and friends. These feelings of gratitude and strength guided me into a career of health. I wanted to be a similar pillar for anyone and everyone.

I never had much interest in food, and mac and cheese is where my cooking talent ends. (And even that is questionable.) I did not consider being a dietitian until a mentor of mine told me that "food makes people sick or healthy." So, armed with my graduate school knowledge of biochemistry, microbiology, food science, health, and metabolism, my professional journey started in 1997. I jumped right in and put everyone on balanced diets, teaching clients about portions, calories, and macronutrients. I was going to *make* them healthy.

And it worked! One of my very first clients lost thirty pounds. Together we reached her goal of lowering her cholesterol and her blood sugar levels, and I felt like a superhero!

And then she gained it all back almost immediately.

I was surprised by her weight gain, but I also felt awful because I had failed her. I wanted to help people find long-term, sustainable health, but clearly, I wasn't doing that. I thought back to the little me that had wanted so badly to help people heal and realized what I'd missed. In the 1980s, there was a department store called Bullock's across from my doctor's office. I remember being petrified of going to the doctor but also, desperately wanting to feel better, so my mom told me, "Don't cry, we can go shopping after your doctor appointment." With that, a shopping addict was born. While my physical body showed up to these doctor appointments, my mind wandered the racks at Bullock's, until eventually I responded to discomfort of any kind with an urge to shop.

The same thing was happening with my client—she was treating food the way I'd treated shopping. It was entertainment or a distraction, or just to feel better emotionally, but food was not just food. Life had gotten unfamiliar—uncomfortable—for her at a lower weight, and neither of us were prepared for what that would mean. My education had taught me all about bodies and almost nothing about the people living inside them.

Remembering the way I had focused on shopping instead of negative emotions changed my practice. Instead of telling people their problems, I started listening to them. I listened to what my clients had to say and saw patterns and similarities during the moments when food became less about fuel and more about fun, comfort, and even fear. Over the next couple of years, everyone from A-list celebrities to middle school students would share similar stories: they'd white-knuckle their way through a restrictive diet, lose weight, get sidetracked, and gain the weight back. I kept hearing about the same issues over and over:

"I eat healthy, but maybe too much."

"I'm a stress eater."

"I feel tired all the time."

"I'm frustrated with my weight."

"I hate to exercise."

"I want something sweet after every meal."

"I can't control myself around food."

"My friend lost thirty pounds on Whole30; why can't I lose anything?"

"If I could just lose weight, I would be beautiful."

Losing weight and keeping it off isn't only about food; it's about your *relationship* with food. And changing your relationship with food is all about identifying triggers, modifying your behavior, and better understanding *why* you eat.

I've studied neuroscience, Western medicine, Eastern medicine, spiritual psychology, quantum physics, psychology, astrology, meditation, and functional medicine to better understand our relationship with food. It has allowed me to develop a method that lets me help people move past their one-night-stand diet plans and short-term flings with food, so they—so *you*—can concentrate on simply feeling better. We're not just trying to shed pounds because someone implied that we would "look better" in a wedding dress or tuxedo, or juicing because our neighbor told us it's healthy. After all, what happens the day after you lose all the weight?

This book and the Kim Shapira Method are all about creating habits that allow you to see lasting results from being healthy and staying healthy. We are going beyond weight loss to weight *maintenance*, to help you feel free around food in a way that allows you to sustain normal eating and your healthy weight without ever restricting yourself.

That's right—this is *not* a diet book. This is for anyone who is sick of dieting. It's for the girls who have become women and still hear, "Are you going to eat all of that?" from their mothers. It's for the men who were bullied in school locker rooms when they took their shirts off. It's for the people who were told by their doctors to lose weight or they would need blood sugar or cholesterol meds. It's for the parents who want to help their children get healthy without crushing their self-esteem, and for the children who are desperate to be allowed to make their own choices. It's for the stressed-out, confused, food-loving, food-hating, restricting, binging, diet junkie in all of us.

We are going to change your relationship with food so that you can be your healthiest self.

UNDO THE TRIGGERS ATTACHED TO FAT, DIET, AND CALORIES

Pop quiz: What does the word "fat" mean?

Is it something we eat? Is it something we have? Is it something we are?

It's shocking how one word can represent so many different things. Fat is fat, but also fat is definitely not fat. I have heard endless definitions for "fat" over the years, but one theme appears again and again: shame. Fat shame is a universal prejudice. As a society we are obsessed with thinness. Burn fat, reduce fat, get leaner, get lighter, and do it faster! We tell each other, and ourselves, that fat means laziness, a lack of willpower, and weakness. Lose it, lose more!

Stop.

Take a deep breath.

We need to redefine this word.

There is nothing shameful about fat—no matter how much or little you have—and telling ourselves otherwise won't make anyone healthier; in fact, just the opposite, as "fat shaming is found to lead people to put on more weight."[1] Talk show host James Corden said it best: "If making fun of fat people made them lose weight, there'd be no fat kids in schools."[2] Instead of bullying ourselves, we need to take back the massive power we've given fat, and see it for what it is: *a vital nutrient.*

Quite simply, our bodies need fat to keep us warm, cushion our organs and bones, absorb vitamins, and serve as a tank of reserved fuel for any future famine or issue we may encounter, like the flu or worse. There is nothing shameful about fat, so the next time you hear, use, or see the word fat, allow yourself to appreciate what it is without allowing a negative jolt to spiral through you.

There is also nothing shameful about the word "diet," despite how the word or your history with diets might make you feel. We equate "diet" with restriction, punishment, and green smoothies topped with flax seed. All of our favorite foods snatched from our hands, leaving us hungry and unsatisfied. Paleo, Atkins, Keto, Skinny Bitch . . . they all tell you what you can't eat. Or worse, they tell you exactly what to eat: Celery juice every morning! Only fruits that start with the letter P! It is hard work to comply with these rules, but you can do it! Willpower! After all, it's only for thirty days, right? Or until your wedding day? Or that beach vacay?

Diet failure is why the diet industry is such a moneymaker. If that last fad didn't work, you move on to the next one. The latest and greatest diet books become short-term bibles that preach a world full of smoke and mirrors. Unattainable bodies are an irresistible siren song when broadcast over social media. If we see something that works for a friend or a celebrity, we want to try it. If it helped them, it could help me. Right?

But here's more trouble: If you put two people on the exact same diet and track how they feel emotionally and physically, you will learn that each person responds very differently. Maybe one person has high cholesterol. Perhaps another has digestive issues. When you follow someone else's diet, you're usually not even eating food you like! You're relying entirely on someone else's likes and dislikes, and when you eat in a way that doesn't come naturally to you, the truth is that we eventually give up. A short burst of willpower will only give you a short burst of results. It is not an unlimited resource.

We are humans with fast-paced lives and short-term memories, so it's only a matter of time before we retreat to our comfort zones and revert to our old ways. When the restrictions stop, the weight comes back. (The worst part? You usually gain *more* weight back than before you started the diet because when you lose weight from a strict diet alone, without taking proper maintenance steps, you're actually losing a combination of water, fat, and muscle. Losing muscle slows your overall metabolism. Not to mention, your body kicks into survival mode, storing more fat than usual just in case you need it.) Yet when what works for that friend, neighbor, influencer, or classmate doesn't work for us, we blame ourselves. And the word "diet" continues to trigger shame.

So, from here on out, diet no longer means a short-term eating regimen. Our diet is a work in progress, a long game that is specific for your body, a flexible plan from day to day and meal to meal that is dependent on your needs. It is not a plan given to us by others; it is a personal lifestyle we create for ourselves.

To create the right diet for our bodies, we must learn to trust ourselves again. Traditional diets teach you how to eat in a vacuum, leaving you stranded when you carefully plan a desk lunch, only to be thrown into a lunch meeting at a restaurant that doesn't serve "approved" food. Or when your neighbor made you a loaf of your favorite bread, just as you swore off carbs. Or a worldwide pandemic shuts down your usual food source. It is easy to get confused and lose confidence in your ability to make food choices when you're relying on inflexible guidelines written by a stranger who has no idea what your day entails. So what I do is provide the tools to make your own choices without panic or time-consuming research. Tools to guide your wellness compass.

Your wellness compass is, as you've probably guessed, just like your moral compass—only for wellness. These compasses are the belief systems you're tethered to. Let's say that we're sitting together at a restaurant when I smile and suddenly blurt out, "I have the best idea!"

You'd naturally get excited as your dopamine receptors light up in anticipation of what I am going to suggest.

Then I whisper, "Let's go rob a bank!"

You deflate, probably laugh a little, because that is not what you were expecting at all. "Oh my gosh, Kim. That's the dumbest idea I've ever heard."

You react that way because your moral compass wouldn't let you rob a bank. But your wellness compass is probably a bit less well calibrated than that—or maybe you're just not used to listening to it. Either way, a sign of a malfunctioning wellness compass is a thought like, "Yes, let's definitely drink that latte with milk even though I am intolerant to milk" or "I will simply force myself to eat celery because I had a cheat day yesterday." The latte and the celery aren't actually the problems here. The problem is we get caught off guard because we don't have conviction in how we eat or why we eat or what we eat.

That is why we're redefining diet as something that we create—that flexes with us and responds to our wellness compass. And to calibrate that wellness compass, I'm going to arm you with a set of six simple rules.† These rules are simple tools that will be your strength when you are wavering in your conviction. You will use them every day. They will start as rules that become habits and then eventually transform into your new value system, something that's as much of a reflex as your response to someone suggesting you rob a bank.

> **RULE #1:** Eat When You're Hungry
> **RULE #2:** Eat What You Love
> **RULE #3:** Eat Without Distractions
> **RULE #4:** Take 10,000 Steps Every Day
> **RULE #5:** Drink Eight Cups of Water a Day
> **RULE #6:** Get Seven Hours of Sleep

Our minds are on autopilot most of the day. We will work on waking up and *changing* that autopilot. While you're learning and applying the rules, you will need to be alert and intentional about why you are eating. But we are *not* obsessing about your food. No more spiraling. No more counting calories.

A calorie, by the way, is simply a measurement of the fuel in our food. According to the Merriam-Webster dictionary, counting calories is defined as "to keep track of the number of calories in the food one eats so that one won't eat too much."[3] But when a relationship is no longer working, do you write down every single interaction you have with your partner in a desperate effort to regain control? No, because that would be bonkers. So stop writing down your calorie intake. Calorie counting takes the pleasure out of eating and makes us

---

† You can think of these as "habits" or "pillars" or "guidelines" or even "things to remember"—whatever helps you internalize them without feeling restricted. I refer to them as rules the same way that a kindergarten teacher refers to "Treat others as you want to be treated" as "The Golden Rule." Think about them more as a rule of thumb than something that's restrictive. Still, I call them rules because, in the beginning, they are not negotiable. They result in weight loss if you need it, lower cortisol levels, less pain, better digestion, and improved blood sugar, blood pressure, cholesterol, triglycerides, mental well-being, sleep, kidney function, and cardiovascular function.

feel guilty for even eating one calorie more than we "should." It might start out harmless, but it far too often becomes obsessive and controlling. It affects your judgment and creates irrational behaviors. Counting calories has been linked to "unintended consequences such as extreme negative emotions, fixation or obsession on your diet, excess competition, and unwanted weight gain."[4]

The six simple rules offer a daily check-in with how your body is feeling and what you need. We need calories every day—but we never need to count them.

Trust me—growing up, my parents never talked about calories, diet, weight, or nutrition. I mean, never! My family's pantry and refrigerator were stocked with everything from chocolate milk, cereal, ice cream, and fudgsicles, to drawers of vegetables, bowls of fruit, and a basket of fresh bread. We were never told no when it came to food, so my siblings and I did not grow up with fears and stigmas around food. We were also never given food as an exciting reward or treat. It was just always available, so I ate when I was hungry and moved on. (On the other hand, we saw others search through our pantry with glee, stocking up on foods they didn't have access to at their own homes.)

Today, I have three daughters, and much like my own mother, I stock our pantry with everything. As a parent, I might say, "Let's wait on a snack so you are hungry for dinner," but if my child asked for ice cream for dinner, I gave it to her—and I never treated it like a special occasion. I just put the ice cream in a small bowl right next to the other foods on the table. I never forced my kids to eat when they were not hungry or made them finish their plates. I did not worry if they didn't eat fruits or vegetables, though I always served two or three at every meal. I put tiny cookies in their lunches every day until they got tired of them. As a result of having free reign over their own bodies, they paid attention to what they needed and what made them feel good.

Recently, one of my daughters told me she couldn't believe how many kids seemed obsessed with their bodies, their weight, and what they could and could not eat. She didn't understand this mindset. I felt that I had achieved a personal victory when she told me, "You know, Mom, fat is not a bad word." That is exactly how I want you to feel as you read this book. We are removing the shame spiral and the fear these words provoke.

WHAT IS YOUR WHY?

Before we get started, let's tackle a big question: *Why* is changing your relationship with food important to you?

What is your *why* for picking up this book? It sounds like a simple question with an obvious answer: "To lose weight, Kim. Duh."

But *why* do you want to lose weight? You might say you want to look your best for a big upcoming event. Maybe a wedding or a trip. Maybe you want to lower your blood sugar or cholesterol. Maybe you want more super likes on Tinder (I've been married for a long time, so ignore me if that's not a thing anymore). Short-term goals like these give you a good jump of motivation out of the starting gate, but rarely do they keep you going after you've lost the weight. They don't provide you with a reason to keep going, so the habits you instill to get there don't stick. Your *why* must be bigger than an event. It must be something that will push you forward for years to come.

Everyone's *why* is different, yet ultimately the same: for peace of mind and a better quality of life. That is what you're really hungry for. And satisfying *that* hunger means getting back the power that food used to have over you.

✎ Start by writing down your short-term goal:

_____

_____

Now, ask yourself *why* you chose that goal. *To have more confidence? To feel good being yourself?* Look at your past, your present, and where you want to be in your future. Your real *why* is your motivating factor when life throws you a curveball. Something you want on your lowest day when it is the hardest to stay on track. *This* is what you are really hungry for.

✎ Take a moment and reconsider your *why*:

_____

_____

Understanding your *why* is like finding the match that keeps your flame lit.† You'll gain confidence when you trade food anxiety for knowledge of what makes your body (not your friend's body) feel its best. The more you make choices aligned with your body, the better you'll feel, so it'll become easy, even fun. I feel good about my decisions, and myself, when I make choices that align with my *why*. My *why* is to feel balanced, so I intentionally and consciously make choices in my day that make me feel that way. I am not perfect, and I make mistakes, but having this intention ensures I lead a more balanced life than if I did not try.

Think of your *why* like this: you're on a journey with me, and you brought along a backpack full of rocks. These rocks are your traumas; they represent your diet baggage, the shame we feel about our food habits, weight, or lack of control. The backpack is heavy, and our journey is up a steep hill. It's hard and you might want to give up before we reach the top, but if a person you love was stranded at the top of the hill and needed you, I bet you would haul ass to get there, no matter how many rocks were in your backpack. We push past our limits when someone else is our *why*, but this time I want you to push out of love for yourself. You're worth it.

Will your *why* keep you connected when your event passes or when you want to disconnect? Will your *why* keep you committed to finding solutions and to taking actionable steps when food seems like it might be more fun than what you are feeling? If necessary, revise your *why* a little and keep it focused on *you*.

_____

_____

Your *why* will be your new superpower, your inner power. It is a new muscle to make that bag feel lighter than ever. Like "paint the fence" or "wax on, wax off"

---

† If you don't have a why yet, don't panic! The stories and info in this book will give you plenty to choose from. Buying this book was the first step toward achieving real inner food power that sticks. Think of all the spare time you'll have when you're confident in the decisions you make about food and no longer spend hours researching the newest fads or stressing about your diet! Just by being here you've proven that you're ready to take back your life from toxic diet culture, and I'm so excited and honored to be your sidekick.

trained the Karate Kid even before he understood their purpose, your *why* will give you the boost to follow the rules even before you have proof that they work.

And, in case you're wondering, you do have to follow *all* six rules. They're more effective when followed together, so you can't pick the ones you like and disregard the rest. But I promise you that if you follow all six rules simultaneously, you will continue to see results. You might fluctuate because of factors like salt and hormones, but you will not plateau. Eating only what your body needs by eating when you're hungry and by being intentional and starting with half of your normal portion will get you more and more in tune with your body's needs. Eating what you love will mean you never need to feel without or restricted, and that leads to sustainable lifestyle changes. Eating without distractions will help you identify how and when you were using food as entertainment rather than fuel, so that you can switch those behaviors. The steps will allow your body fat to decrease along with your weight, while the water flushes your system and proper sleep keeps your body in homeostasis. Altogether, the process works because it allows you to see that food is simply fuel and improve your metabolism.

THINK IT. WANT IT. GET IT.

This book is brimming with things that will help you on this journey. We will talk about the medical theories and facts behind my six rules. Every chapter is loaded with helpful anecdotes from my clients, tips, tricks, insights, advice, reminders, everything I've done throughout my long career that has helped people lose weight, keep it off, and maintain a healthy relationship with food. What are the most common pitfalls? What gets people stuck? What gets them unstuck? It's all in here, including Taking Action boxes that will give you concrete strategies to implement. My goal is for you to say, "It's easier than I thought it was," and for you to realize you have everything you need inside of you to survive every moment of every day. You are going to define your own boundaries. You will take control of your relationship with food without allowing it to consume every thought. You will have food freedom. You will know what hunger is and trust that there is more food later. Your food will be satisfying and will be food *you* love, not what I love. And lastly, you will see food as fuel and eat cake, too.

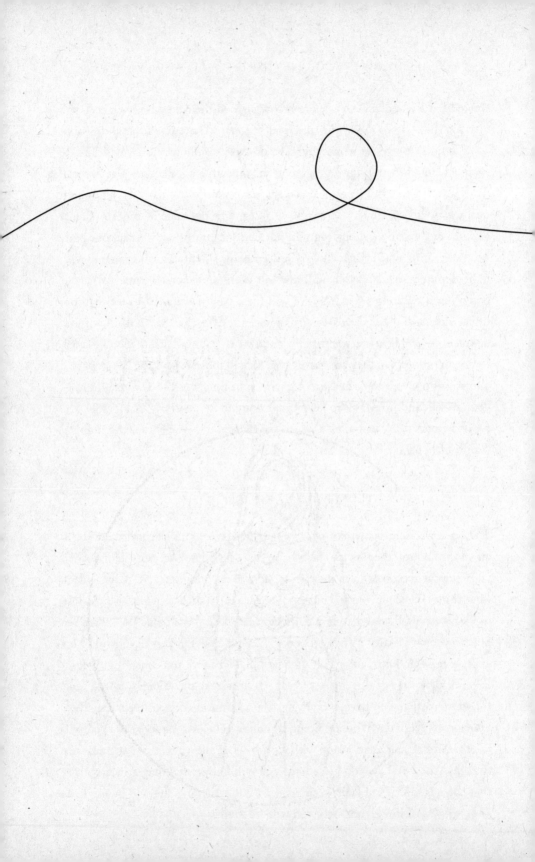

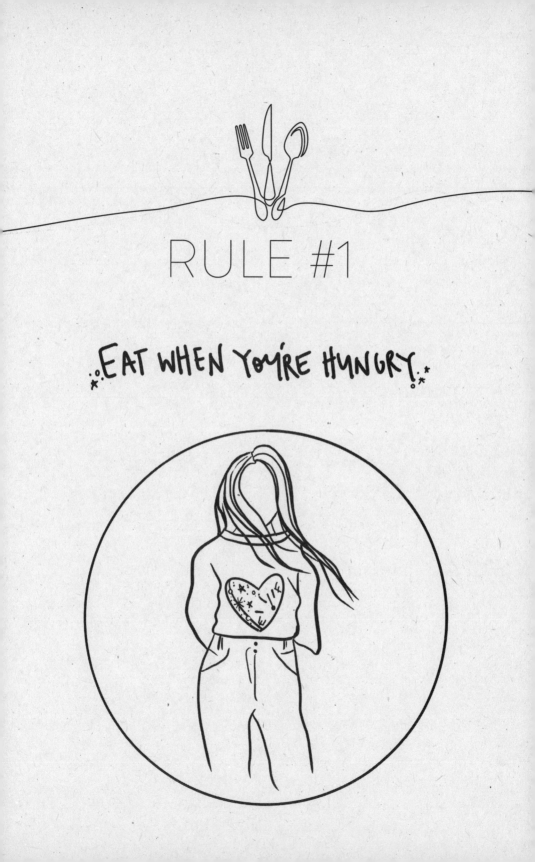

RULE #1

EAT WHEN YOU'RE HUNGRY.

EAT WHEN YOU'RE HUNGRY—YOUR BODY IS TALKING; ARE YOU LISTENING?

We need to eat. And we need to do it when we're hungry. I know this sounds silly and simple, but it's neither, because most people have never been taught to eat when they are hungry. In fact, many people I've met view hunger as a negative thing. Some will say it's annoying, uncomfortable, painful—scary even. But 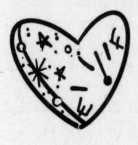 hunger is just a physiological response to your body needing food. It's a sensation in your stomach—a series of muscle contractions often called hunger pangs (*not* pains) that can get more intense the hungrier we are—that is there to remind us we need to eat. (Yes, even in our society with food on every corner, and meetings centered around food, we need this basic reminder to let us know that we're ready for fuel.) The point of hunger is to make it impossible for you to accidentally starve to death—to let you know that you need more energy from food.

Food has vitamins, minerals, water, carbohydrates, proteins, and fats—all nutrients that we need to have balanced, healthy, thriving, comfortable bodies. Eating when you're hungry means that you're eating when your body is actually primed to properly absorb those nutrients. All the enzymes, hormones, and neurotransmitters associated with digestion are ready for action. Because of that, eating when you're hungry helps balance your blood sugar and regulate your weight.

There are a lot of feelings or sensations our bodies create, but the feeling or sensation we get for physical hunger isn't that different from the sensation you get when you feel like you need to use the restroom or when you know you are ready for bed. These all involve your body sending a signal to your brain to say, "Hey, pay attention to me."

Let's use the example of needing to use the restroom. We all just kind of know when that time comes up, right? You don't stop what you are doing and think, *Hmmm, interesting. My bladder is signaling to my mind to alert me it's time to think about finding a bathroom.*

What actually happens is that you get an alert, and then your mind scans your body. In a matter of seconds, you have determined if you need to jump off a Zoom call, or if you can wait for the show you're watching to end. The whole time this assessment is happening, you are able to engage physically and mentally with something else. And before that Zoom call or TV show—before the day even started at all—I doubt you woke up and thought to yourself, *Hmmm, I am going to have to pee about six times today; I am going to plan my day around finding a toilet.*

But a lot of people do plan their day around meals, despite the fact that hunger is similar to needing to go. First, you can't always plan when you'll be hungry. If you're eating because you scheduled yourself to eat, you may be ignoring hunger signs. But just like there are bathrooms everywhere, there are often food sources everywhere, on every corner, in every city. The worst that can happen if we don't plan out our meals is we get too hungry—just like our bladders could get too full. It's uncomfortable, but sometimes not preventable. Second of all, even if we don't plan our days around mealtimes, we've still often been training ourselves to eat for other reasons besides a hunger signal, like for comfort, boredom, stress, or fun. We created misfires in our mind and our body when we ate without being hungry, and when we continue to act on them, we turned that behavior into something automatic.

The way to break those habits and start to eat when you're hungry is to be aware of what you're actually feeling when you think that you want to eat. The next time you find yourself searching through the cabinets for a snack or sitting down for a meal, pause and ask yourself *why?*

Please don't answer this right away. Think about it first. I often talk about progress over perfection. When we strive for perfection, we end up getting stuck and frustrated, so we quit, postpone, or never start at all. And the unnecessary stress of this affects our bodies, our momentum, our plans, and our progress. If we are striving for the perfect time to make a change or start eating better, we will keep putting it off until tomorrow or the next day, and we end up wasting precious time, leading to high stress, burnout, and anxiety. If we strive for progress, we are at the least getting started. Seeking progress allows us to find and foster ways to promote positive experiences. It allows us to begin to see each moment, snack, or meal as an opportunity to enhance our lives. Aiming for perfection can make us inflexible and critical, while seeking progress can make us openminded and curious. And when you think about why you're eating, you can really find progress. So think about it on your way to eat and while you are standing around eating; think about it after you eat.

Progress might look like thinking about food and recognizing you are not hungry, and so letting the thought pass. Or maybe you make your way to the kitchen and find something to eat, and, as you are about to dig in, you realize you aren't hungry, so you save it for later. Progress can even be eating a few bites and realizing you aren't hungry, so you stop. If you are aiming for perfection, though, it can feel like as soon as you miss the moment you started eating and you eat, you have failed. It can be so hard returning to a new habit once this happens, because it's not perfect, so what's the point? Instead, approach your journey from a place of progress. And do *not* treat thinking about why you're eating as a form of punishment or shame; the purpose is to bring self-awareness into the moment you are in.

Sometimes I catch myself right as I am about to have a sip of coffee. I knew I needed water, so why did I reach for coffee? When I am in that moment, I can recognize that it's because it is habitual, it tastes delicious, and it's a single hit of fun. Then in that same moment, I might say to myself, *I don't actually need that hit of fun; I am okay.*

So why do you eat? There are four reasons why we eat:

1. We see food.
2. We are emotional.
3. We have a craving.
4. We feel actual physical hunger.

We make 221 food choices every day.[1] A food choice can be as simple as water or coffee, salt or no salt, fish or chicken; or as complex as how much food we need in this moment, or if we can wait a few minutes or hours before we eat. But we frequently consume food that our bodies don't need because we're making food choices based on the first three reasons. We aren't physically hungry; we aren't in tune and listening to what our bodies are really trying to tell us. So let's break down these reasons:

Reason #1: We See Food

Close your eyes and imagine getting into your car. You open the door, slide your right leg in and then your left, and shut the door. You turn on the engine, adjust your mirrors, put the car in reverse, and back out of your driveway. The crazy part? You probably don't think about any of those actions while you take them. You just do them. You might have a spot on the floor where you always put your bag. A turn that you always take on your way to work. You don't have to think about setting down your bag or making that turn. This is called autopilot. (The average person spends about 46.9 percent of their day on "autopilot."[2])

Now, close your eyes and imagine yourself walking into the kitchen. What do you do first? Do you fish through your pantry for a snack? Do you go directly for your favorite treat? How do you eat? Are you standing? Are you chatting with family members? Are you on autopilot?

We eat in our kitchen so often that our minds are usually no longer engaged in making choices about our meals. We help the kids with homework or watch Netflix while our hands feed our bodies without us. Suddenly, we wake up and realize we've finished a whole bag of chips without noticing we were eating them.

How many times have you been at a party and caught yourself snacking on shrimp cocktails or mini hot dogs without even realizing that you were doing it? I call this type of autopilot-eating the "see-food diet." When we see food, we eat it. When we walk by the kitchen on our way to another room and stop to pop something into our mouths—that's what I call "walk-by eating" or "fishing."

Think about Thanksgiving. It's just dinner on a Thursday night. We could eat that food any night of the year—but we stuff ourselves simply because the food is there, everyone else is eating, too, and it's an annual event. How about Halloween? When the house is suddenly filled with candy? That's stressful for many people, yet that same candy is available at every single store 365 days a year. It's everywhere. You can have it whenever you want, but suddenly, when it's right in front of you, it's so much more tempting. Why? Studies show that the average American gains weight between October and December,[3] but we aren't any hungrier during those months, are we? We're just eating because the food is in front of us.

Reason #2: We are Emotional

If your child walked into the room and said, "I am so stressed," would you say, "Oh, let's go eat! That's what I do, and it works for me"? No, you would say, "It's okay to be stressed; it's going to pass. Let's try taking a deep breath; let's try talking about it or going for a walk." Would you tell a child to eat instead of cry when their hamster dies? I hope not. You would tell the child that the feeling will pass and try to help them cope another way.

But oftentimes, we don't give the same grace and good advice to ourselves. Emotional eating can be complicated because different emotions will cause different reactions in each person. Maybe it's boredom, fatigue, stress, loneliness, fear, anxiety, or really any emotion. But whatever the emotion, emotional eating happens when our minds tell us that food is more fun than what we are

feeling. It is a trained behavior. We are such a habit-dependent, automatic spe-
cies, and our bodies seek consistency—even if the consistent behavior is hurting
us. Our minds' job is to help us survive in the most pleasurable way. And if we
found comfort or joy in eating and it numbed discomfort in the past, a habit
was formed.

The good news is we can train it away. A thought to eat that was triggered
by an emotion will pass when the emotion passes. And since we are emotional
people, we get new emotions often. According to Harvard brain scientist Dr. Jill
Bolte Taylor, "ninety seconds is all it takes to identify an emotion."[4] The entire
wave of emotion from identifying it, to labeling it, and then to accepting it only
takes ninety seconds. If we can sense and identify the emotion, then we can
address the real problem. And usually, the impulse to eat simply stops becoming our first impulse. Progress here might resemble being aware of what your
body is feeling when you think food is a good idea—acknowledging that an
alarm might be going off, but scanning your body to see why rather than simply
responding. Because, while the discomfort that hunger causes us will always be
fixed by food, unfortunately the discomfort our emotions cause will not be.

I was supposed to meet with my new client, Margo, for the first time,
but it just so happened that I was also experiencing a rather chaotic day. I was
working from home, managing a sick kid, and being forced to rearrange my
schedule because the plumber showed up at the wrong time. Everything was
totally out of whack, and I was running late. Margo was right on time. She was
well dressed, polite, and ready to lose sixty pounds. The session, regardless of
my personal turmoil, got off to a good start.

The problem was that I kept getting interrupted. We were running out of
time, and since I had another appointment directly after, that meant Margo
would leave our first session without a plan. That would have driven me nuts, so
I did something that I had never done before: I asked her to return later in the
day when I had more time. Luckily, she could fit it into her schedule. She was
going to meet her wife, eat lunch, and then come right back.

I asked her, "What do you plan to have?" (She did not know this was a
leading question.)

"The same thing I always have. A margarita, chips, and guacamole, and two tacos."

I could tell immediately that this order was automatic for her. She wasn't scanning her body to tell how hungry she was—or even if she was actually hungry. It was clear to me that, rather than being about physical hunger, she was eating because food was a way for her to connect with her partner.

So I told her, "Great! Go enjoy your partner's company. Skip the cocktail, try one taco, and I'll see you in a couple of hours."

She let loose an audible gasp, fear radiating off her. I've seen that expression many times. It's the visual that everyone gives when a voice inside says, *I'm going to be starving because that's not enough food. I can't do that!*

"Trust me," I told her. "There's only two hours between now and when we meet again."

Despite her fear, she agreed because she was eager to succeed. She'd been on so many diets that any challenge around food immediately sparked a sense of competition. As a result, willpower that she'd relied on to muscle through new diets kicked in. Willpower won't get you through the type of changes that will lead to sustainable health. It's way too easy for the spark of pleasure that we feel when starting a new challenge to be replaced by the pleasure that comes from caving to a taco habit—and then to ultimately give up because we feel weak and ashamed. In this case, though, I was counting on her "willpower" to be enough to get her through this one meal and give me the opportunity to retrain her brain right off the bat.

Sure enough, when Margo returned, she reacted the way most everyone reacts when they first try to go on any diet. "I'm starving," she told me, holding her throat. This was exactly what I expected.

"Where do you feel hunger?" I asked.

She was confused by the question. She looked at me like I had asked her what planet she lived on. "In my throat."

"Hunger is in your stomach. It's not painful. It's not scary. It's not uncomfortable," I told her, because the feeling or sensation Margo felt in her throat wasn't hunger. What she felt was something else entirely.

By holding her throat, she was telling me that, for her, eating wasn't about fuel. She was telling me that this meal and her food was about fun and joy, mixed in with quality partner time. And maybe even some fear of what her partner might think or feel if Margo didn't eat or drink. To be clear, I am not saying that Margo only needed one taco that week or that she needed one taco every week. It's natural for us to have an emotional connection to food. We should have pleasant memories around food. We should love the food we eat. And we should also be able to connect to when, what, and why we eat. So what I am saying is that Margo needed to be flexible and listen to her body to hear how much she needed. No one's needs can or will be the same on every Tuesday.

TAKING ACTION

Take a moment and write down for yourself: What does food make me feel? (Some examples are *happy, comforted, scared, annoyed,* or *bored.*)

 Do I eat because I have a need for fuel?

_____

 Does my hunger come out of nowhere or do I notice it grows stronger over time? (If it shows up suddenly, that's usually an indication that it's not hunger so much as a need for comfort.)

_____

 Answer quickly and without thought: What do I use food for?

_____

_____

> ✎ Take some time and answer this a bit more thoughtfully: What is food for?
>
> _____
>
> _____
>
> ✎ Can I make food simply one important part of my life, like water and sleep?
>
> _____
>
> ✎ Can I practice connecting to my emotional self before I start eating and noticing if I need fuel for my body or am I seeking a feeling I think food gives me?
>
> _____

Reason #3: We Have a Craving

Cravings are not hunger! While we typically feel these urges physically, they are different from physical hunger pangs. Sugar and salt withdrawals are a pulling, a need, a nagging in your body, in your hands, in your mouth, in your head, or in your chest. But cravings *do not* happen in your stomach.

For some people, one bite of sugary food tips off the pleasure receptors in their brain, giving them a positive feeling. This gets stored in the brain, and whenever their body needs another pleasure hit, it remembers sugar.

When we eat sugar, the sensation is so pleasurable that our brains have to adjust to tolerate it. As a result, the brain releases a large amount of dopamine. Dopamine is a neurotransmitter that our bodies make in the nucleus accumbens (this is the same area of the brain that responds to addictive drugs). It allows us to feel pleasure, satisfaction, and motivation.[5] The brain's reward system activates, linking sugar and dopamine. When we repeat the activation of this system, our brains adapt. This means we need to eat more to get the same rewarding feeling.[6] We experience physical symptoms of withdrawal when the receptor is communicating to our minds that it wants more hits of pleasure.[7]

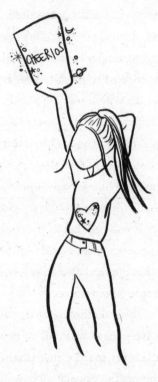

Plus, our brains make their own version of opioids, called endogenous opioids. They are chemicals that act just like opioid drugs; they attach to receptors in your brain and they help your body experience sensations of well-being and control pain.[8] Endorphins are one form of endogenous opioids. Our body releases endogenous opioids when we fall in love, when we laugh, when we exercise, among many other things, but it's important to note it's also released when we eat sugar.

Most people have no idea the effect that sugar has on their body. But to resist cravings of this sort, we have to stop our body's natural response to indulge. If any of you have tried, though, you might have noticed that we can develop withdrawal symptoms that can be quite unpleasant but thankfully lessen over time. Withdrawals are why some people feel like they need sugar in their bloodstream to feel better, if not normal. But that is an illusion—or "seduction" might be a better word. I know it is because I was one of those people.

For most of my life, I would eat a Butterfinger or some Chips Ahoy! cookies on a daily basis without thinking twice about it, but after my third child, I was breastfeeding and exhausted all the time. With a new baby, I expected I would be exhausted—but then one of my friends declared that it could be the chocolate milkshake I was drinking (or maybe the tons of Oreos that I was also inhaling . . . my chocolate cravings were intense when I was breastfeeding!).

There was no way that I would give up chocolate. No way! So I refused to believe my friend could be right. A life without chocolate is not a life at all. I didn't want to know that those cookies could have been what was sapping my energy and making me tired. I thought up all kinds of excuses, but my friend had planted a seed and my science-loving mind got curious. After throwing my mental temper tantrum, I pulled myself together and decided to conduct a little experiment to see if the sugar was the culprit. I was going to give up sugar for five days. That was my plan.

Before I even made the promise to myself, I was already in the kitchen, scrounging around through the cabinets looking for some kind of sugar. Anything! I could feel that craving everywhere in my body. There was a pulling sensation in my arms—one that I had never noticed before because I had never stood still long enough to acknowledge it.

It was bad, but in the back of my head, I knew that it was not hunger I was experiencing, so I held out. For the next couple of days, I was bitchy, irritable, and in physical discomfort, but I didn't give in, though I had access to any sugar I could have wanted.

Then, on the fourth day, the cravings disappeared. Nothing changed in my house—sugar was still everywhere in multiple forms, but some kind of peace came over me. I didn't want chocolate. I didn't need chocolate. I wasn't even tempted by chocolate. I'm serious. I even forgot about the experiment and went on with my life.

Without even realizing it, sugar had taken a back seat. A few weeks later, Halloween rolled around, and the house was filled with more candy, but I still wasn't tempted to eat any of it. In fact, I was indifferent. For the first time in my life, I was able to clearly see candy for what it was. I looked at the plastic coating on the chocolate and had no desire to put that in my mouth. I am not saying I never eat it; I just don't see it the same. I feel empowered, and saying no doesn't feel like I'm denying myself (which is the same way I know you will feel around food after you finish reading this book: calm and peaceful).

A few months after Halloween, I was throwing a party at my house, and casually talking to a group of people in the kitchen when, without thinking, I happened to pop a macaroon in my mouth, in a move that was purely part of the "see-food diet." I didn't think anything of it and probably would have forgotten I even ate it, but the next day I found myself back in the kitchen, scrounging through the cabinets for chocolate.

Recognizing that as a craving was enough to get me to walk away, because I knew it was temporary. That "aha moment" for me was awesome. I saw how the pieces fit together. I had the choice to either eat the chocolate or see it as a craving. I knew that I wasn't going to die either way (yeah, my thoughts were that drastic), so I walked away. When I did, I took with me some power and a new posture that said, "I got this." I had shown myself that I could eat a cookie if I wanted to, and I could walk away if I wanted to. This whole interaction with myself lasted only a few seconds.

I'm not sharing this story to imply that you can't have sugar (more on that in Rule #2). It's normal to have candy or something sweet occasionally. Just don't succumb to the seduction of snacking on any food, sugary or not, when you aren't actually hungry. Sugar is an anytime food, but it's not an all-the-time food. So once you have the thought to eat and can almost feel it in your mouth, label the thought.

Then, take a second to scan your body: Are you hungry in your stomach, or do you just want something fun in your mouth?

If you just want something fun, remember your *why* and put the sugar on hold. It will be there when you really are hungry, and your body needs fuel. Try to follow these simple steps when you want to eat something sweet:

1. Feel it.
2. Acknowledge it.
3. Laugh at it.
4. Leave it alone.

I know what you're thinking: *Yeah, that sounds great, but it's never that easy.* But . . . maybe it is. Eating normally, without restricting yourself or slipping into a dieter's mentality, means sometimes eating whatever sugary thing you are thinking about. But if you're eating something every day or every night at the same time, that's not eating normally—that's giving into a craving. That is a habit, but it's one you can break. You can walk away from any food at this time, even if you never have before. And remind yourself that it will be there later or tomorrow when you're actually feeling a hunger pang. (Though, fair warning, more times than not, if you put the food you are craving on hold and walk away, it's very unlikely it will be what you want when you are hungry, so you might find yourself eating less sugar.)

Jake was a client who claimed he was an excellent dieter. He was enthusiastic about losing weight. He loved the competition of it all, the planning, the drama. My biggest challenge was going to be replacing his joy and excitement over losing weight with some joy and excitement about the comparative monotony of keeping it off. (Where I wanted him to find peace, he was seeking a roller-coaster ride.) The trick was to get him to see that he was going to gain more joy and lose the burden and weight. I did know that he would be really good at following the rules, though, even though he had a history of binging, because he approached the world in a very black-or-white, on-or-off way.

He lost thirty pounds right away. Then Christmas hit. During Christmastime, he was around so much candy that he couldn't help himself. Every day at work he was gifted chocolate; the same thing happened at all the parties he attended. His enthusiasm with those chocolates was tempting him to pause the journey—he was thinking that he'd hit his goal, lost thirty pounds, and now he could give up on the rules for a little while. His mind was being hijacked by sugar and the excitement of it in his life.

Since we could predict this trigger, we focused and set intentions. He just needed to recalibrate and regain his balance—to show the candy who was boss. So I told him, "Just eat it. Make it your meal. You can't gain weight if you're eating the chocolate when you're hungry." I know, and I think you know, that most people, when given the choice, don't choose chocolate when they are hungry. For a variety of reasons, most people save it for after they're full from something else, treating it like a reward for eating. So he needed a reminder that it was okay to eat—that chocolate is a food like any other. This took away the need to binge by helping him realize it wasn't going anywhere and that he could eat it and still maintain his weight loss.

It worked. Soon after he allowed himself to eat the chocolate for his meals, he realized it wasn't satisfying. Then he started seeking other types of food. The candy became less important, and, when he would feel a pulling in his hands or chest, he recognized that it wasn't in his stomach. He wasn't hungry. Jake didn't give up sugar; he made it part of his life. And since this led him to see how some of his actions were not aligned with his goals, he has been able to maintain his weight loss without ever restricting himself.

Now, salt cravings are a different story. Our bodies are designed to like salt because we need sodium to survive. Sodium is the mineral that controls the proper balance between minerals and water. If the fluid balance in your body starts to fall below what is healthy, you may crave salt. And when you have too much salt in your body, your brain is stimulated to make you thirsty; then you drink more water and create more urine, so your body can rid itself of excess salt. (The body regulates its salt and water balance by not only releasing excess sodium in urine, but by actively retaining or releasing water in urine.) Sodium actually has a starring role in the body's health: it maintains normal blood pressure and is essential for nerve and muscle functioning. So, to be clear, *salt* is actually a crystal-like chemical compound—sodium chloride—and is abundant in nature, while *sodium* is a mineral component of sodium chloride. In other words, we do not technically need salt as long as we have sodium daily to replace what we lose through saliva, sweat, urine, and feces.

If you are craving salt, it could be that your body is dehydrated, bored, or stressed, or your body may not be able to retain salt well, such as with adrenal fatigue. You may crave salt if you are working out harder, longer, or in extreme heat. Hormone fluctuations also cause water imbalances that can cause salt cravings. Some of the symptoms you may have from sodium deficiency are confusion, headache, loss of energy, drowsiness, muscle weakness, bloating, low blood pressure, spasms, and/or nausea and vomiting.[9] Occasionally wanting popcorn or chips isn't unusual, but if you find yourself constantly or suddenly seeking out salt, it's definitely worth a trip to the doctor because it could be linked to a medical condition.

But while our bodies absolutely do need sodium, the average person is consuming much more salt than they need. Too much salt can lead to an increase in thirst, affecting blood pressure and causing bloating and poor-quality sleep. If you feel swollen or have tenderness in your chest, you may be ingesting too much salt. And, just like with sugar cravings, we don't want salt cravings to trick us into eating when we're not hungry. It's worth starting with a full glass of water or two, and waiting a few minutes to see if you are actually hungry or just thirsty. When you find yourself wanting something salty, wait until you're hungry to eat it.

Another common craving people have is for ice—which can be more concerning than you realize. Maybe you think, *Nah, I just like it*, but craving ice can be a sign that you need to have your iron levels looked at. You can have an iron deficiency because iron is a difficult mineral to absorb. If your diet is high in cheese or milk and low in animal protein, if you take calcium supplements, or if you are in the habit of using products like Tums or Prilosec, you might need more iron. Our bodies use iron from our diets to make hemoglobin, which is the protein that carries oxygen from our lungs to every part of our body. So if you find yourself craving ice (or perhaps even dirt or clay) or experiencing extreme fatigue, brittle nails, fast heartbeat, lightheadedness, and even a change in your skin tone, please reach out to your primary physician or dietitian instead of continuing to just crunch on ice.

When Buddha said, "Life is suffering," he was right. Choosing to fight cravings can feel like the worst kind of suffering. Cravings can be intense, and at the time can feel like the only thing that matters, especially when you think you love what you're craving. Your mind will come up with all kinds of excuses and justifications for why you can eat that food. When you're in the midst of a craving, you have seductive blinders on—so to stop suffering, you have to find a way to remove those blinders.

Think back to last week. Do you remember any of the food you craved, or even ate, for that matter?

That food may have seemed like the best thing in the world at the time because our minds whisper that eating it is so much better than not eating it. But just like the feeling you experience when you have to use the restroom, it will pass—and be quickly forgotten. The next time you experience a craving, try not to focus on the food you want; focus on what's making you think you want it, and, if it's not hunger, put the food you think you want on hold. Eat it once you know it's hunger in your stomach.

TAKING ACTION

Don't ignore the sugar craving—challenge it! If you are one of those people who struggle with cravings, conduct an experiment. Distract yourself every time you have a craving for five days. It will be hard. It might suck. You will want to eat that food more than ever before because your brain will be screaming at you to ease the withdrawals, and you're going to want to give in, but promise yourself that you can have sugar, candy, ice cream, cake, or whatever you want when you are hungry after the five days. Just see what happens.

After a few days, those receptors that are causing you to crave sugar will no longer be functioning. You might surprise yourself when you find that once those little receptors stop communicating, you won't want sugar. Giving this up doesn't have to be permanent; this is an experiment. Just be open-minded. You do not need to be perfect, but this does only work if you give it a few days, so if you end up eating sugar before the five days are up, just start again without getting upset with yourself. Are you curious if sugar is seducing you?

But what if I really, really want it? Well, no two people have the exact same feelings, and some might have a more difficult time resisting cravings and urges than others. I get it. It's hard, but we can do hard things! The most important thing to remember, though, is not to replace the food you crave with other food, even if it's "healthy."

Clients come to me all the time, asking why they can't just eat something "healthy" every time they have a craving for a chocolate bar or a cookie. The reason is that a craving is not hunger, and you don't want to eat when you aren't hungry. Your body doesn't know or care whether the food you eat is "healthy." If you aren't hungry, then your body doesn't need the food and will store it as fat. If you aren't hungry, then trading out a food you want for something else is a form of restriction. And restrictions aren't sustainable. Most people just end up eating what is "healthy" . . . and then also eating what they really wanted.

Reason #4: We're Physically Hungry

When your body needs more fuel, you should eat.

Early in my career, I was interning at a weight-loss clinic in Boston, working with folks who weighed over four hundred pounds. They were doing a shake diet to lose weight. Back then, I had so many irrational fears around food, like that I needed to eat first thing in the morning or I would pass out from starvation. But I was curious, so I decided to skip my cereal one day and try the shake they were drinking.

I think I lasted less than thirty minutes before I felt hungry again. So I ate food, surprised the shake didn't hold me over. How was I so hungry so soon after drinking it?

When I got to work that day, I asked multiple participants how they were managing on the shake. Every single one of them was confused. They ate because it was time to eat, because it was more "fun" to eat than not to, or maybe because the food was in front of them, so the shake was just what they had to do as part of this program. It had nothing to do with how they really felt.

We aren't taught what hunger is—we don't even talk about hunger itself much at all. We focus on calories, good food, bad food, breakfast, lunch, and dinner, but we don't focus on hunger being natural and the body's sign that it needs fuel. No one teaches us that food isn't a reward but a necessity.

If a person isn't physically hungry, do they need food? And if they don't need food and they choose to eat, where does that food go? It gets converted to fat, because the body is amazing and efficient. If you are eating when you aren't hungry, you're telling your body that you're planning for a famine, so it needs to store this fuel for the future.

That starts a cycle in which we stop getting hungry but we eat anyway, because we expect to or we think that we're expected to. Maybe we went fishing in the pantry but had a lunch on the books, so we ate both times. Maybe when we're hungry doesn't quite match when our families are, so we eat again when we're with them. Maybe we think we need to eat, even though we're not hungry yet, because we don't want to be starving during a one-hour meeting that coincides with our typical lunchtime.

But to *stop* doing that and start eating for reason #4—when we're hungry—we have a bit more work to do.

✳ 2 ✳

EAT WHEN YOU'RE HUNGRY—THROUGH THE LOOKING-GLASS

When I was growing up, my dad would always say, "You can lead a horse to water, but you can't make it drink." That saying didn't make any sense to me. *I* could make that horse drink! And when I started working with clients, I didn't want to believe the saying was true. Doesn't everyone want to be healthy? We all know the consequences of overeating and a poor diet. Nobody needs me to tell people that, right?

Wrong!

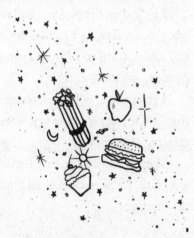

For years, I watched most of my clients leave the office convinced that they would be able to understand themselves and their actions when it came to food—but then it would all go out the window in the moments they needed that knowledge most. Why is something that seems so obvious, that people know will benefit them, so difficult to do? Many people are excited to join a gym in January but quit by February. I know these same people are looking for the next best thing and really want the change they thought a gym membership or a diet plan was going to give them. I was perplexed.

Until I realized that we're all distracted. Our schedules these days are insane. We all have complicated lives. Over the course of the average day, we're pulled in different directions. We have short attention spans and forget. It's easy to feel overwhelmed and stressed. During those moments, our brains go into autopilot and revert to our old habits. It can happen so fast that we don't even realize what's going on. We simply slip into past behaviors because they're comfortable. That's how we trained ourselves. It's like a reliable, good-for-nothing friend who keeps showing up to borrow money from us. The first step to resetting these habits is being able to identify the state that we're in.

I have always booked my clients back to back. One thing about me is that I hate running late. If I am behind schedule, I run the risk of upending everything else. Years ago, if my clients were running late, I would use those moments to eat, thinking, *I am not sure when I will have time again, so I better do it now.* (This was one of my "food issues" or trained behaviors.)

Around this time, I was at home sitting in my living room. My phone started ringing—but this was before cell phones, so I actually had to get up and go to the phone hanging on the wall in the kitchen.

I picked up the phone—and really wished I hadn't. The person on the other line was a talker, and I didn't have the time for it right then. But this landline had a long cord, so before I even realized it, I found myself walking with the phone to my pantry.

I remember, as I was looking for something to eat, thinking, *How strange that I am in front of my pantry, when a second ago I was in my living room not really thinking about food.*

Then it dawned on me: I was feeling the same way I did when my clients were late. I was anxious. I had unwittingly trained myself to eat during times of anxiety.

"It's a poor sort of memory that only works backwards," remarked the White Queen to a confused Alice in Lewis Carroll's famous book *Through the*

Looking-Glass.[1] Alice had just told the White Queen that she can only remember things that happened in the past. The Queen is blown away that Alice's memory only works one way, and suggests she try to remember things from the future.

I believe we can all see how our weeks play out—we can see the future. Based on our history, we know exactly how our week will go. If we don't understand how or why we repeat our actions, we will keep making the same mistakes. I know exactly how my client's week will go if they do not change, and if we are being honest, you also know exactly how your week will go if you decide to ignore your history. Referring back to our discussion of progress over perfection at the beginning of this book, this is a good time to implement progress. Forget perfect; strive for better than you did before.

THE RATIONAL BRAIN VERSUS THE IRRATIONAL BRAIN

When we are calm and grounded, our minds are in a rational state. When we get triggered, our brain flips out and becomes irrational. Our rational mind tells us that food is fuel, and we should get in shape and stay in shape because it will keep us healthy. Our rational minds tell us that we want to maintain a weight that will help prevent disease.

But it's still so hard for us to do what we all know to be common sense because our irrational mind takes over and convinces us that chocolate tastes so good, it's okay to eat it now; we can worry about health tomorrow. Our irrational mind tells us that it will be more fun to sit on the couch, eating pretzels and watching television—we can start exercising next week. To give into temptation and engage in behaviors that we know will make us feel bad later. It's so powerful that it can cause a grounded, rational person to do irrational things and rationalize bad ideas.

When I first meet with a new client, I ask them to answer two fill-in-the-blank questions—and I want you to do the same thing. Technically, it's actually the same question, but the first time I ask them—and you—to answer with the rational mind and the second time answer with the irrational mind. I want people to understand the difference between their rational mindset and their irrational mindset. Though even this is putting the cart before the horse, because 50 percent of the time, when I ask people to answer with their rational mind, they still answer with their irrational mind because they can't recognize the difference.

Fill in the blank: "**Food is** _____."

When people answer with their irrational mind, I'll get responses like:

"a party."
"fun."
"good."
"comfort."
"always there."

Some people will go so far as to say:

"bad."
"horrible."
"something that makes me fat."

When answering with their rational mind, people give answers like:

"fuel."
"nourishment."
"a necessity for survival."

To move through this process, you need to think of food as fuel and nourishment—as necessary for you to be alive. You need to prevent your irrational mind from hijacking the plan and blinding you to reality. To do that, you must identify your triggers.

IDENTIFYING YOUR TRIGGERS

Everyone has triggers; it's a human thing. We are emotional beings. A trigger is a person, place, thought, event, or feeling that activates our irrational brain, causing us to act on habit and become experts in rationalizing unhealthy behavior. We all have triggers that prompt us to hide, numb, self-soothe, and cope. When I used to get triggered, every emotion would tell me go shop for fun. Now I know I'm not feeling okay (or I have been triggered) when I think, *I want to go upstairs, get in bed, and read.* Even though that's much healthier, I can't go read a book in bed at 3 PM. It's still a sign that I need to breathe, check in with my body, and most likely delay the gratification. I do this all of the time, and the moments pass. Some of you get triggered and think food is a great idea. Whenever we get triggered, it is lightning fast—but we can get great at being aware of the lightning.

Everyone has several areas of sensitivities, hot buttons, sparks, or activations that can potentially set them off. Most of these hot buttons are formed in the first six years of our life, but it doesn't mean we had bad parents or a major trauma. We all have triggers, regardless of what our home life was like. Triggers are like soft spots that became permanent wounds—like repetitive stress injuries. It is amazing that years zero to six are the years that shape us, and yet also the ones we least clearly remember.

As children develop, their early "emotional experiences literally become embedded in the architecture of their brains."[2] This time period is when we develop the ability to understand feelings and emotions. We recognize the way we feel and the way others feel, and hopefully we develop healthy ways to manage those feelings. When we experience trauma, we develop new hot buttons. Think about COVID-19: none of us are coming out unaffected, yet we all have and will continue to have different experiences.

Every day a part of our mind, the prefrontal cortex, is doing its thing, reasoning, creating, and problem-solving for us, while another part called the amygdala—which is not rational—is casually going about its day detecting threats. Enter an unexpected spark of something we are sensitive to, and we totally flip out because when our amygdala detects any threat from something we see, smell, feel, or hear (the news, a comment from a friend, your child's anxiety, taxes, the wrong dressing on your salad, or anything else), it takes over. This makes it very difficult to make thoughtful choices. Whether the threat is real or not does not matter—our brain and our body cannot tell the difference. We just react, leaving trapped energy and emotion that our mind perceives as discomfort. Our mind then will find a way to end our suffering, so it will default to how we found pleasure the last time we felt this way. For many folks that form of pleasure comes in the form of food or alcohol. Then we eat and drink without recognizing that we've just added more rocks to our backpacks.

We can't predict how we will be triggered.[3] What we can do instead is understand and appreciate our bodies' responses and learn how to remain unaffected.

TAKING ACTION

Let's look into how your body responds to a trigger. Write down the last three times you ate mindlessly. Think about this time; close your eyes; picture your body—can you sense what your body was feeling? Do you remember what was happening around you?

My bet is you had a feeling in your body that was telling your mind, *Food is more fun than this feeling.* Can you connect the dots to this feeling in your body and the thought to eat? Once you realize how and when you rationalized eating when you were not hungry, you can recognize what your body was really trying to tell you.

I know that one of my triggers is fairness. This trigger, like any trigger, takes me right out of the moment I am in. I get anxious. My mind immediately starts seeking ways to make a situation fair to everyone involved. I find myself in my head solving this "problem" while others are completely unaffected. One example of this trigger affecting me is at dinner parties, even the ones I'm not hosting. I'm always overly concerned that everyone has a good seat, that they can hear everyone, and that they are comfortable. It's just ingrained in me. But once I was made aware I was acting this way—though it took me a minute to see it—I accepted it. Being aware of my reaction helps me stay grounded and lets me laugh at myself. I can't make everyone comfortable—it's up to them to advocate for themselves. I'm still helpful, aware, and doing my best in the moment, but I don't burden myself with the worry or angst that can build up to the point where I become untethered from my rational thoughts.

My client Grace lost her husband of thirty years five years before the pandemic. Her kids are grown up, so she sold her home and moved into a condo. She started visiting one of her sons and grandchildren frequently to cope with the loneliness, and they soon made it an everyday event. On her way home, she would always have the same thought: *Chocolate sounds really great*. So she'd stop at the grocery store to buy some, eat a few bars in the parking lot, and then be upset with herself for overindulging.

But it wasn't the chocolate that she craved: she was triggered, and stopping to buy and eat the chocolate let her delay returning to her new normal without her husband. The candy bar was not only a more pleasurable experience than the ache she felt in her heart, but, because she was ashamed and full of self-loathing after eating it, she never had to deal with her grief—she was too busy beating herself up.

I asked her to go ahead and buy the chocolate—but to wait to eat it until she got back to her kitchen table. What I was asking of her might sound simple, but it wasn't easy. I was removing her security blanket. I wanted to give her another option, a different way to view her daily experience. She thought the chocolate was the problem, but the chocolate was a shiny object blocking her from seeing the real problem.

At first, there were some days when she would make it home, walk in, and forget about the chocolate. Other days the chocolate was all she could think about. But days of forgetting about it turned into weeks. The daily binges petered out to occasional temptations on random days every so often. The chocolate lost its appeal when it stopped giving her a chance to hide away.

As human beings, there is no way to remove pain or discomfort from our lives. There will always be times when we need to be comforted—but when we identify we have been triggered and are able to see that we're eating because of that sensitivity and not because we are hungry, we can stop using food as comfort. We often underestimate our ability to respond differently.

I have a thirteen-year-old client who was fifty pounds overweight. They are one of the smartest kids I know. They are a gamer, winning almost every chess match they play. Keeping their brain occupied is a challenge. Every time we approached my six rules, they felt genuinely sad, defeated, and restricted. I wasn't getting through to them.

We were chatting one day in my office when they mentioned their obsession with horror movies. BOOM. I had a way in. They pulled out their phone to show me a clip from Stephen King's *It*. A scary clown approached a little girl with a birthmark on her face. (I was already scared, but I wasn't about to let this kid know that.) The girl told the clown that she couldn't talk to him because he was a stranger. The clown offered to remove her birthmark. The little girl lit up! Forgetting her stranger-danger training, she asked for the clown's beauty expertise. (Ugh! The mom in me was shaking.) Long story short, the clown ate the girl. Terrified, I assured my client that one clip was enough. I also used this as a teaching moment.

I told my client to think about food as if it were the clown. Food is trying to tempt us when we know we're not hungry. Instead of giving into irrational thinking like the poor little girl in the movie, we have to be the hero in our own story and stand our ground. We have the strength to tell things that are getting in the way of our success to hit the road. We eat food—it doesn't eat us!

Once you can identify in your day the moments your mind flips into threat mode, you can begin to practice training your mind and body to remain unaffected. Having a greater awareness of what sets you off will allow you to manage the moment and reflect on what your body really needs. And most of the time, what you need is a deep breath. The type of deep breath that says, "This moment will pass, and I have everything I need in me to survive until it does."

WHEEL OF FORTUNE

If you have a history of failures when it comes to keeping weight off, or feel shame in seeing your doctor for an annual appointment because you haven't lowered your cholesterol, you might be overwhelmed and confused about where to start. I am going to give you a visual guide to help you connect to a balanced lifestyle while keeping your focus on *progress*. Because nobody is perfect. (Repeat after me: nobody is perfect.) Perfection is a trap, and traps are restrictive. We all have strengths, and we all have weaknesses—and we all need to find ways to better connect with these different aspects of our lives to become well.

There are seven areas that impact the balance of your life. To be and stay well, we cannot neglect any of these important areas. I've found it useful to think of those seven areas as making up a wheel—a Wellness Wheel.

The seven spokes on our wheel are:

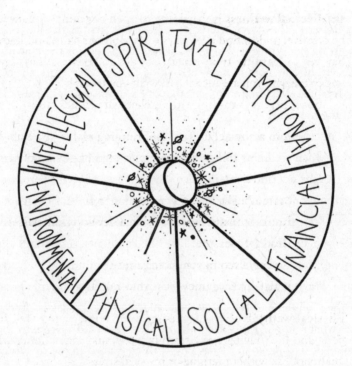

1. **Emotional wellness** is the ability to cope with life in a healthy way while creating and maintaining healthy relationships.

   Some practices to help with emotional wellness are:

   - Check in with yourself and acknowledge the way you feel. It's okay to have all the feels in your day. This check-in will also help you see that you are stronger than you think.
   - Start a self-care routine. Carry aromatherapy with you and take deep breaths often. Work on calming your body and your mind throughout the day.

- Be honest with the way you feel. Say no when you need to say no.
- Seek out support groups, family and friends, or a mentor if you feel lonely. Look into employee assistance programs.

2. **Intellectual wellness** is the ability to open our minds to new ideas, to be creative, and to find new ways to expand our skills and knowledge. Say yes to learning from others, say yes to conversations, say yes to understanding you are more than what you thought.

    Some practices to help with intellectual wellness are:

    - Join a book club, fan club, running club—any club. Make a list of things that are interesting to you and research to find a group.
    - Start a hobby you always wanted to start.
    - Look into ongoing professional development classes.
    - Read for pleasure.
    - Get involved in your community.
    - Journal, play games—use your mind.

3. **Physical wellness** refers to moving your body, eating well for your body and life, having good sleep hygiene, and maintaining a healthy quality of life without fatigue or physical stress.

    Some practices to help with physical wellness are:

    - Start a movement routine. Plan for it. Schedule it. We are working on progress, so add a little more every day. There is no rush as long as every day you work on it.
    - Find a friend to keep you accountable, to try new workouts with, and to keep you motivated.
    - Eat what you love when you are hungry. (More on this in the next rule.)
    - Set an alarm to remind yourself to go to sleep, remind your mind it is sleep time—not solve-the-world's-problems

time. Wind down and work toward going to sleep at the same time consistently.

- Set regular doctor checkups.
- Rest—set time aside each day to do nothing.

4. **Spiritual wellness** is the spoke that refers to your beliefs, ethics, and the values that guide your life so you can maintain peace and harmony. This is where you might explore opportunities to engage with your purpose and meaning in life.

Some practices to help with spiritual wellness are:

- Become part of a community, either virtually or in person, that shares similar values or beliefs.
- Start a gratitude practice: either via texting with friends, quietly to yourself first thing in the morning before you use your electronics, or in a journal, make sure you find three things every day you are grateful for.
- Carve out five to ten minutes of uninterrupted time to practice meditation.
- Practice random acts of kindness in your day.

5. **Social wellness** is the ability to establish and maintain strong positive relationships with family, coworkers, and friends while also creating time and space for adventure.

Some practices to help with social wellness are:

- Schedule activities that you can look forward to with friends such as pickleball, playing cards, a book club, or vacations.
- Train for a bike tour, hike, or a marathon with a friend or group.
- Engage in activities that are low stress and high joy.
- Have friendships that allow you to have healthy boundaries.
- Remove notifications on your electronics and delete apps and social feeds that stress you out.

6. **Environmental wellness** means taking care of your personal surroundings as well as living in an environment that supports well-being.
Some practices to help with environmental wellness are:

   - Declutter your workspace and living space. Get organized,
     and create spaces that help you have positive emotions.
   - Spend time outdoors. Find ways to add more natural light
     in your day. This helps your mood, your sleep, and your
     stress level.
   - Consider gardening or composting.

7. **Financial wellness** means being satisfied with your current and future
finances.
Some practices to help with financial wellness are:

   - Understand your own budget.
   - Seek financial advice, take classes, read a book on planning
     for the future.
   - Plan your finances. Create an emergency or rainy-day fund.
   - Find little ways to save money during the day to contribute
     to your rainy-day fund.
   - Don't feel guilty over spending money on something you
     really want. Instead, consider putting that item on hold
     and walking away, kind of like the fifteen-minute trick. It
     will be there when you return.

Study the Wellness Wheel and consider how connected you are to each
spoke. Taking stock of where you are in each area of your life can help reveal
vulnerabilities and areas where you can improve. That's important because those
low areas could be what's triggering you to eat when you're not hungry. Once
you notice that some of the important parts of your life have been neglected,
you start to see why food has become more than fuel. When we connect to what
brings us real joy, food is less likely to be a source of joy.

TAKING ACTION

Study each spoke of the Wellness Wheel, and rate how connected you are to each spoke, with 1 being very little and 10 being deeply connected.

Emotional	1	2	3	4	5	6	7	8	9	10
Intellectual	1	2	3	4	5	6	7	8	9	10
Physical	1	2	3	4	5	6	7	8	9	10
Spiritual	1	2	3	4	5	6	7	8	9	10
Social	1	2	3	4	5	6	7	8	9	10
Environmental	1	2	3	4	5	6	7	8	9	10
Financial	1	2	3	4	5	6	7	8	9	10

Check in with the wheel weekly to stay connected to what is truly important to you. Start small by making daily adjustments in each spoke. Be realistic, and know that if you miss connecting with something on a particular day, it's okay. We have a long journey ahead of us—and it's not about the destination. It truly is about finding joy and connecting while you progress.

TAKING ACTION

Picture yourself. Now take that image and make it two: your physical body and your emotional self. Think about how many times you asked your heart to beat today, or your lungs to breathe, or your stomach to digest, or your mind to think. My guess is there were zero times. Your body did it all without you doing anything. Kinda cool. So basically, our emotional selves live inside and are sheltered by this amazing self-regulating, self-healing, fully functioning body. I feel grateful that my body can do these things. And all it needs from me is to respect it, honor it, show it grace. Our body has a language—and we know it without even knowing how we know it.

DISSATISFACTION IS NOT HUNGER!

One client told me that when she went out to lunch with her friends, she didn't like the salad she ordered. She picked at it and ate some of the bread on the table. When they were done, she decided that she "didn't really eat," so she felt that she still "needed lunch."

If it was hunger, of course she should have eaten more! But she wasn't hungry; she was dissatisfied. I agree her meal wasn't satisfying, but that doesn't mean that it hadn't satiated her hunger.

As you practice, you will learn to recognize the difference between dissatisfaction and being hungry. Dissatisfaction is not comfortable, but the feeling will pass—and you probably won't remember the meal you were dissatisfied with in the long run. When your mind tells you it's okay to eat more, you will need to check in with your stomach to see if you are really hungry or just not satisfied. You experience discomfort in many ways throughout your day. Discomfort is holding your bladder or being thirsty. It would be great if you could get by without any of this, but really that discomfort is just telling you what is happening in your body. Remind yourself that you will get to eat again.

TAKING ACTION

Take out a piece of paper and write down all the feelings you typically feel when you eat when you are not physically hungry. Write "_____ = eat" and fill in that first blank with things like being tired, stressed, bored, anxious, excited, annoyed, grumpy, lonely, and so on. Once you have your list, erase "eat" and fill in those blanks with something else. Something you would tell your loved ones to do if they felt this way. Use your Wellness Wheel (see page 40) to connect to what is important to you.

An important part of the process is treating yourself properly, and learning to accept the moment that you are currently in. Jon is forty and has been a binge eater since he was ten. His father is an alcoholic, and the compulsions are similar. He drinks nine Sprites a day. He often gets up throughout the day to have a sip or two and then goes back to what he was doing.

What is actually happening here is that when he gets bored, his brain senses discomfort and tells him that there is something fun two feet away, so take a break. That lights up his dopamine receptors. Those pleasure sensors tell him that a sip of soda will help him get through those next few moments of being bored.

But if you're bored, you first need to accept that you're bored. Next, you have to wait it out, or find something else to do without turning to food. We all have boring tasks, but you can find other ways to make them more enjoyable without abusing yourself in the process. Just keep reminding yourself that it will pass. We are not going to like all of the moments we are in, but still, stay in the moment; don't let your mind wander. You will get better at this skill with practice. When your mind does wander, and you do bring it back, you are actually training your mindfulness muscle. Connect back to your Wellness Wheel, plan some fun, bring balance that might be missing in your life, and help those uncomfortable moments pass a little faster.

Take Stock of Your Mind and Body

When you think, *Food is a good idea right now*, stop what you are doing and ask yourself, "Why am I thinking about food right now?" Then do this practice: Ask, "Where is my body?" Then notice your body is right here. Then ask, "Where is my mind?" When we actively ask this, our mind goes and looks for itself. It's really cool. We can track our mind, which is a great trick to practice. This practice will help you notice if you flipped your lid at some point and will allow you to ground your mind back in your body so you can make a rational, thoughtful decision. If food is fuel, we eat it when we are hungry.

Often, the best way to take power away from a feeling is to acknowledge its existence. It only takes ninety seconds to identify an emotion and allow it to disappear.[4] If you can ride out the rough wave for ninety seconds, you might not even remember that you wanted to eat. Also consider the idea that you can put food on hold until you are physically hungry. It's not going anywhere and, more likely than not, you can always get more tomorrow.

If you can't tell if you're hungry or not, don't eat right away. Stand still. Wait ten minutes and reassess. Take a deep breath, recall that your mind is in your body, and put a space between the thought and the action to eat. Feel your feet on the ground. Let the moment pass and use that moment to figure out why you want to eat. Is it because someone else is in the room or at the table? Are you really hungry, or are you just bored? Did you just get uncomfortable on a phone call? Did you see someone who makes you feel sad or angry?

The more you check in with yourself and the more you make it a habit, the more in tune you will become with what your body is telling you.

TAKING ACTION

Take thirty seconds now to watch and label your thoughts; this simple act will come in handy for the rest of your life. Close your eyes: view your thoughts as they pass in your mind. Don't engage; do not think. Simply see the thought and label it as positive, negative, or neutral. Notice what happens once you label it. It disappeared, right? This practice trains your mind to stay in this moment.

When you become more mindful of why you're eating, it's much easier for you to develop normal eating habits. If you're obsessing, counting, or measuring food, you are not eating mindfully. What you need to do instead is see the thought that *food is a good idea* as just an alarm. Label the thought and stand still. It was only a thought and is temporary. Acknowledging the thought is the point of being mindful.

Sometimes we are just in a funk, and our brain tells us that food is more fun. In those cases, try setting a timer for thirty seconds, and, during that time, smile as hard as you can. See what happens. Try it again. Keep repeating it. Only good things can come from this. Smiling in stressful moments tricks our bodies into relaxing; it helps by lowering blood pressure and our heart rate. Smiling releases mood-enhancing hormones that help with pain and stress.

Smile therapy is fun. You can also listen to high-vibration music (if you're not sure what I'm talking about, google it), or listen to positive affirmations. I have done many of these things; they may seem silly, but they actually work.

If you aren't sure whether what you feel is physical hunger, try drinking a glass of water and waiting fifteen minutes. Some people think they're hungry when they just need water (we'll have much more on water in Rule #5). If you're not hungry, whatever you were feeling will usually go away after drinking water. Using water to slow down eating is helpful because it "wakes" your mind from autopilot and helps put space between the thought to eat and the action to eat. Plus, if you are experiencing physical hunger, the feeling in your stomach won't go away, so you'll know it's really time to eat. You can also consider making your water fun. Add lemon, lime, mint, or cucumber. Drink it out of a straw or make it warm. There are lots of options here. Drink up!

Another thing that you can do when you're not sure if what you're feeling is hunger is find a scent you love and carry it around with you. Our nervous systems are the only systems in our body that we can control. In our fast-paced lives with triggers everywhere, we might need assistance keeping our feet on the ground and our minds in our bodies. If our minds are off saving us from future problems, we can't really scan our bodies to see if we are hungry. Aromatherapy is a natural way to help us regulate. Take out the scent and try to inhale as slowly as possible. That slow inhale is like a hug and a massage at the same time. Try doing it five to ten times; I can guarantee you will be more relaxed than you were before you started. And then scan your body to see if you are actually hungry.

YOU HAVE EVERYTHING YOU NEED INSIDE OF YOU TO SURVIVE THIS MOMENT

When you look back at your history, you can say that you have survived every moment of every day so far. You can channel that to survive future moments.

Imagine you have a red balloon full of air attached to your body by a string. Once you are triggered, the balloon starts to rise. Slowly or quickly, it starts to pull away from your body. If you are unaware it is happening, you won't be able to feel what your body needs, because the balloon is floating above you. It's your job to notice the balloon has left your body and to reel it back in. We can call this practice "grounding." This is the training you have to commit to that will lead to a more trusting, confident, peaceful mind.

Remember, emotions can change in ninety seconds. They are like clouds floating by, and we need to trust that the sky is blue behind every cloud. Knowing a feeling is temporary makes it easier to ride out the uncomfortable period until you return to the rational mindset. A few hours later, chances are you won't even remember that initial negative emotion because there can also be moments of joy and peace thrown in.

To help you better understand, I want you to close your eyes and think about what it feels like to be fairy royalty, like from a children's movie. Everyone is in awe of you; they love, respect, and think very highly of you. Everyone wants to be you. How do you feel when you are this person? How do you carry yourself?

Now, erase that image and think of a new one. This time you are the smelly, sinister swamp villain. People cross the street to avoid you and never make eye contact. How does it feel to be in that body? How is it different from being that most beloved person? Which one makes you feel better?

Pay attention to how your mind has a thought and your body reacts to that thought. Did one make you feel tall and floaty while the other made you feel small and ashamed? All of those feelings began with just a thought. Sometimes, you can change your mood and outlook by simply thinking of something else. When you find yourself in a negative headspace, try to think of something that you love. This will change your body chemistry and help you relax.

✳ 3 ✳

EAT WHEN YOU'RE HUNGRY—SLOW AND STEADY (IT'S NOT A RACE)

Okay, so you know that you're physically hungry—you listened to your body. You put some yummy grub on your plate and then scarfed it down.

The problem?

You stopped listening to your body as soon as you picked up your fork. You didn't notice when your hunger signals stopped. A few minutes later, you're feeling bloated, tired, and stuffed instead of energetic and satisfied.

Your brain and stomach operate on one system. As you eat, your stomach sends information about the food entering your body to your brain. However, this is not an instantaneous message—it's dial-up. (And if you're too young to know what dial-up is, ask about it the next time someone is telling spooky stories around a campfire.) It takes fifteen minutes for your stomach to communicate to your brain that it is full. In other words, once

your stomach is satisfied, it takes fifteen minutes for that message to reach the mind and for you to recognize the feeling. People often even go back for seconds in under fifteen minutes because they don't feel satisfied, not realizing that they might actually already be full. And even if you're not getting a second helping, if you shove a meal into your mouth as quickly as you can, your stomach doesn't have enough time to say, "Stop! That's enough!"—meaning you could be giving yourself more food than you need.

The solution is to slow down—use the fifteen-minute trick: split your meal in half; eat one half and then wait fifteen minutes before you take another bite. This will give your brain the time it needs to decide if you need more food or if you should save the rest for later. If, after fifteen minutes, you don't feel satisfied, slowly eat more, checking in with yourself after each bite to see where you fall on the hunger scale (see below).

THE HUNGER SCALE

In life when an alarm goes off, we most likely stop what we are doing and scan our surroundings. We need to do the same with the hunger alarm. When we get a thought that *food is a good idea*, we need to immediately pause, see that our alarm is going off, and scan our bodies. Think *wake up*, and make sure your mind (the red balloon from the last chapter, page 48) is in your body. Then you need to scan your body and confirm this thought came to you because your stomach needs food. (It takes a split second, such as when you think you have to use the restroom.) Otherwise, you can easily be off to the races, not understanding or trusting that food will always be there.

And food has always been there, right? It's just like the toilet in that you always find one but don't need to run to the bathroom when you first feel the need to go. The key is to understand that just because you think food is a good idea doesn't always mean you are hungry—just like having half left on your plate doesn't mean you need more. It could be that you want more, or you don't want to waste the food. Each of these thoughts can trigger you, and that discomfort could be enough to drive your mind to tell you it's okay to eat more. We need to be present, in the moment, alert, and intentional. Starting with half

often causes us to feel fearful. We instantly think, *Half won't be enough.* But if
you remember the "wax on, wax off" idea, you'll remember that sometimes you
need to practice without knowing why. To trust this process, you need to jump
in and put this into practice. I am not sure if half of your meal is enough and
neither are you. But if you assume you know that it's not enough, then you are
disconnecting from your Wellness Wheel. I need you to be open-minded. If
you skip this part, you aren't paying attention to your hunger levels.

I know it might be difficult to pinpoint the difference between "hungry"
and "hungry enough to eat," so let's break it down. Next time you feel the hunger alarm, rate your hunger and satiety on the following scale (1 to 10).

ONE (1) Starving:

Food is the only thing you are thinking about; your energy is low. You
might feel weak (your body needs blood sugar). It's an exaggerated sensation in your stomach; it may feel hollow, grumbly, empty—and it will
get worse over time. Your desire to eat is strong. You're feeling threatened.
Your body is screaming at your mind, "Find food now!" Think of it like a
full bladder moment. In addition to feeling tired and weak, you might feel
irritable and cold. You experience serious discomfort.

Unfortunately, you waited too long to eat. Sometimes it can't be helped.
You need to eat, but I still want you to start with half of your normal portion while also trying to think, *It's okay; I won't remember this discomfort
later. It will soon pass.* Just because you are starving does not actually mean
you need to eat everything in front of you. Although sometimes it does.
The goal is to be flexible. Being at a 1 still requires you to stay intentional,
even though you may be hungry enough to eat everything in your fridge.
This is a moment to trust yourself. Since the reality is probably that you
don't need as much as you "think" you do.

To be clear, I am not okay with being starving; I don't think anyone
is. But please still trust yourself—and me—in this moment. I remember
one day coming from a spin class and meeting my girlfriends for a few
hours of Mahjong and lunch. I was starving, ready to eat, ready to pass out,
I was so hungry. I ordered a bowl of tomato soup. It came quickly, like I

had hoped it would. I scarfed it down in forty-five seconds. (Not my finest moment.) My friends' lunches hadn't arrived yet. I was still hungry, but I knew I wouldn't know for another fourteen minutes and fifteen seconds if I needed more food. I decided I would wait and then get more if I needed it. Those waiting moments were uncomfortable, but I was hoping that the soup would catch up with me. I distracted myself with my friends, trusted the process, and, before I knew it, three hours went by before my stomach signaled to me to find food again.

This will admittedly be a lot easier if you can keep yourself from getting to a 1, but sometimes that's not possible. And unfortunately, it will still take about fifteen minutes for your mind to catch up to your stomach, so practice eating slowly, reminding yourself there is more.

TWO (2) Very Hungry:
Your stomach is growling; you are beginning to get antsy and a little desperate. Your stomach feels hollow—you need food, and you are in the beginning stages of that feeling of being at a 1. Your mind and body make you feel this way so you can survive. Just remind yourself that food is right around the corner. And when you do eat, take it slow. Take your normal portion, meaning the portion you would have normally put on your plate, and immediately cut it in half. Chefs have a standard serving, and boxes even have food labels with portion sizes. None of these are *your* portion.† Understand that the second half is available to you in fifteen minutes if you still need it.

THREE (3) Ready for a Meal:
I like it here. This is a great place to eat. You may have a few hunger pangs, but your energy and mood are still good. You are still even keeled. This stage is just an alert from your body telling your mind, "Let's find food." It's been a few hours since you ate—which is exactly where you want to be.

---

† A normal portion is what you normally eat in this situation. An example might be pizza: if you normally eat three slices, start with one and a half. Another example might be roasted chicken, mashed potatoes, and sauteed vegetables; cut all three in half and start there.

Getting hungry every few hours means our blood sugars are balanced. If we get too hungry, our blood sugar takes a huge dip, which creates a ton of stress in our bodies, making our thoughts hyper-focused on reducing stress (in this case, hunger). For us to lose weight and maintain our weights, our bodies must feel safe. Think back to the way our bodies respond during a threat—they hoard. If you are not hungry after a few hours, it is a message from your body that your last meal's portion was more than you needed. If you can get and stay consistent, your body then will feel less threatened and will actually give up stored fat because it knows it doesn't need it anymore.

Take your normal portion and cut it in half, trusting that your second half is waiting for you if you need it, but also acknowledging you will be eating again in a few hours.

FOUR (4) Feeling a Bit Peckish:
Stage 4 calls for snack-like portions. Eating at this number is good, too. Yes, you still need to cut your snack in half because this is the fail-safe way to make sure that you're not overeating. In the beginning, as you are just getting reacquainted with your stomach, try to eat small, frequent meals when you're feeling at a 4 on the scale. Staying around here in the beginning can help you as you gauge how much and how often your body needs food. Starting with small snacks or meals ensures you will feel hunger sooner rather than later, which is the goal: to feel hunger and then to *eat*. I do not want you to stay hungry, as this will threaten your body and mind, and your body will then store food as fat because it will think it is preparing for a famine.

If you can eat a small snack here, I promise that your body will respond by speeding up your metabolism and making you hungrier in the future. That's important because it means your body is functioning properly. Getting hungry means your engine is running. Remember, though, when you're at a 4, you are ready for a snack, not a meal. Trust you will be eating again soon.

From day to day, you may be hungrier at some times than at other times, because our eating patterns change from day to day (no matter how consistent our routines may be). Our activity also changes from day to day, as does the amount of sleep we get and any hormonal shifts. With your body in constant motion, is it really any wonder hunger levels can vary? I've asked you to see being at a 4 as needing a snack-like portion because it serves an important purpose: if you gloss over this level it could advance you straight to a 3, 2, or 1. Snacks are really useful in helping us keep our blood sugar even, which will help us stay intentional so we can start with half.

FIVE (5) Thinking About Food:

If you're eating at this stage on the scale, it's emotional eating—the walk-bys, fishing, or the see-food diet I discussed in chapter one. This is you wandering into the kitchen to drink lemonade or wine, or grabbing a hand-ful of "healthy" nuts, crackers, chips, or cookies. This is you standing at the pantry, staring inside. Or grabbing candy from your office-mate's stash.

Try putting it on a plate to save it for later and walking away. Can you delay gratification, trusting it will be there when you get hungry? Emotions are sneaky, and we have lots of them every hour. Let's not let a passing emotion take us off our journey. So this is a moment for you to really shine. If you cannot tell the difference between being hungry or not, do not eat. Emotions pass, and food does not fix them.

SIX (6) Satiated:

Satiated means satisfied. Eating took the edge off, and now you find you are interested in other things around you. Maybe you are thinking about a book, TV, work, or checking your phone. You are done eating for now. When we are at a 6, we're not interested in food in the same way; it becomes boring. Sure, it would still be delicious, and it would be fun to eat, but we are nourished. Being at a 6 ensures you will be hungry again in a few hours.

SEVEN (7) Comfortable:

You're a little more than satisfied; maybe the food was really good and you just wanted one more bite. It's normal for this to occasionally happen; it's more of a bad habit if it happens after every meal every day. Because while you might still feel comfortable at this point, it's important that you are able to recognize that if you ate more, you would feel uncomfortable, bloated, and full.

EIGHT (8) Full:

We have all been here. I see this a lot when folks are dining out and haven't eaten enough during the day, so they are starving when they start dinner. Or maybe their friends ordered food and they didn't think they could say no. It happens; the goal is not to keep going there. Remember, it's normal to sometimes eat more than we need.

If you reach an 8, you may not reach a 3 or 4 on the scale for many hours. Practice being respectful to what your body is saying—allow it to cycle through the meal, and be patient, waiting for it to give you clues to eat again. But I am not here to reprimand or persecute you for eating too much, and do *not* shame yourself. It happened. Perfection is a trap, and there's never a need to beat yourself up about being anywhere on the hunger scale. If you don't like the way you feel at this point, remember it the next time you are about to eat past satisfaction. The goal is to learn from your history, not repeat it. What matters is what you do next. Get right back to consistency. Go right back to eating when you are hungry and starting with half.

NINE (9) Change-Your-Clothes Full:

Stage 9 means you're so full that it's difficult to focus. And all you want to do is take off the clothes you are wearing because they feel too tight. So this is overeating; this is ignoring your body's needs. And this too happens at times. But you want to avoid it because this will cause your body to think you are trying to store for the winter. This stage can happen because you have been restricting yourself, or because you got distracted while you were eating, or you like the feeling of fullness. I get that; being full is sometimes described as being hugged tightly. If you frequently find yourself at a 9, ask yourself if you're eating because the food is in front of you or if there is some emotion driving this activity—what is this fullness doing for you? And how else can you obtain this same effect, but in a way that may be more aligned with what you really need? Look back at your Wellness Wheel to see where you might feel disconnected, and reconnect.

In the meantime, in addition to always starting with half, when you do eat, try taking smaller bites, chewing more, and drinking water between bites. Give your brain a chance to catch up to your stomach in as many ways as possible.

TEN (10) Thanksgiving Full:

I often refer to this as Thanksgiving full because I think some people give themselves a pass to overeat during Thanksgiving—and that's what a 10 feels like. You experience discomfort as your stomach is stretched past its normal capacity. When it stretches, it pushes against other organs, adding to the feeling of discomfort. This also makes your organs have to work harder and impacts your sleep. Although this is not a permanent feeling, you want to avoid this level of fullness.

The good news is that it's temporary. Just go back to respecting your body and what it needs. You may not need to eat again for many hours. If you trust your body, it will signal when it is time to eat again.

You want to avoid reaching either end of the scale because both sides can make you feel out of control. I want you to be able to decipher the difference between being a little hungry and a lot hungry; between being fulfilled and being full. This hunger scale will help you translate your thoughts so your body can function to its full potential. Overeating and undereating disrupt your circadian rhythms, making it harder for your body to feel safe. Finding the balance of what you need and when you need it allows your body to heal, regulate, and be well.

While I would love for you to eat when you're between a 3 and 4 and finish around a 6 or 7, the real goal here is learning to trust yourself—to know that you will always eat again. Remind yourself that if you feel compelled to break Rule #1 and eat when you're not hungry. It will take a little time, but keep at it because thinking in terms of the scale and documenting how you feel will help you better understand your body, physical hunger, and how much food you need.

Keep in mind that we aren't eating to prevent being hungry later. We *want* to be hungry later. Remember you might still feel hungry after waiting fifteen minutes, and if you are, it's okay to eat some or all of your second half. That hunger means that your body needs it. The best gauge for how much to eat is simply how physically hungry you are. Your hunger isn't always the same. Sometimes you need less (like when you're at a 4 on the scale); sometimes you need more, so allow yourself to be flexible with food.

Though, let's be honest—in the beginning, this might be really uncomfortable. If you're struggling with the waiting time, try to do literally anything else. I'm pretty confident that if you walk away and get distracted, you will forget about the other half or quarter of food you left behind until your stomach reminds you it's time to eat. We really have short-term memories.

But sometimes, it's just going to come down to your *why*. Practice intentionally eating until you are satisfied (a 6 on the scale) and see what happens. After the initial discomfort passes, you might even find it becomes no big deal. The fear of eating only when you are hungry and starting with half is just a rock in your backpack. It goes away as you continue this journey. Don't take yourself off course. Allow yourself to practice.

TAKING ACTION

Forget about counting proteins, carbs, and fat. At this stage, it's not about any of that and it won't be ever again. Right now, all you have to do is get in the habit of checking in with your body, so you can identify physical hunger. Start right now and try to train your brain to recognize why you eat. It might take a little while to identify what your body is trying to tell you, but the more you do it, the better at it you will get.

Trusting the Fifteen-Minute Trick

The idea of eating less than you're used to can feel scary, like a threat, as if that half portion automatically won't be enough food or we are going to starve. But just like we have to use the restroom more than once a day, we have to eat more than once a day. We can't fit all the food we need for the day into one meal any more than we can survive on a single bathroom break. So, since we have to eat more than once anyway, this becomes more about trust. Trust that half will be the amount of fuel you need in this moment; trust that there is more in fifteen minutes; and trust that you will be eating again. You might be shocked to find that by starting with half, you weren't as hungry as you thought.

Let's discuss your normal portion. This is the amount you normally would eat. Not what the label says (which is just there to show you the breakdown of vital vitamins, minerals, and other nutrients inside that food for whatever amount they're calling a portion) or what the restaurant serves you (which they make the same size for *everyone*). Do you usually eat three pieces of pizza, order a large salad for yourself, eat two eggs for breakfast with two pieces of toast and two pieces of bacon? Then that's your normal portion. It's how much *you've* been consuming in one sitting.

Whatever that is, I want you to cut it in half and put that other half on hold. You want to get curious and learn how much food you actually need. We are looking for you to eat to a 6 or maybe a 7 on the hunger scale—a place that lets you get physically hungry so you can eat again when you need to.

Starting with half helps you develop trust within yourself. It will give you confidence that you are in control and you know how to listen to your body. It allows you to align with what you really need—because I'm telling you to start with half, not that you have to stop at half. We are putting space between the thought to eat and the action to eat. There is more food when you need it.

And, as I mentioned, slowing down is half the battle. However, if you've developed the habit of eating fast your entire life, slowing down can be much easier said than done. You'll need to rig the game, or at least level the playing field, so it's a fair fight.

Start by practicing new habits. Put food on your fork, and then take a little off. Put some in your mouth. Put your fork down. Chew your food. Think about your food. Enjoy what is actually in your mouth, keeping your mind from thinking about putting more food on your fork for the next bite. Take a sip of water; use your napkin.

While you slow down, you're learning the differences between *your* hunger levels. My portion is different from your portion. I don't know how hungry you are and what your body needs. Only you know this; you just are out of practice in paying attention.

Flexibility with what, where, and how much you eat teaches you to trust yourself around food—which is what is going to allow you to make your weight change sustainable. After all, one day you could be eating lunch at home, the next on the beach in the South of France. If you ate half of a burrito yesterday and it was enough, that's fine—but it might not be enough today or it might even be too much today. The rule is to eat when you're hungry—not to only eat the same thing whenever you're hungry.

Does a five-year-old need to eat off the adult menu at a restaurant? Do you need the same amount of food as an NFL player? Absolutely not, but . . . maybe. Each meal is different from the one before. Yesterday isn't the same as today. Your appetite is determined by:

- ✦ your level of activity
- ✦ your muscle mass
- ✦ your height and weight
- ✦ your bone density
- ✦ your hunger levels
- ✦ your health
- ✦ your temperature
- ✦ what else you ate today

Your needs aren't the same as everyone else's. Always start with half of your normal portion; stay connected to this in all of your meals and snacks at home and even when you travel. You'll quickly real-ize that your portions won't be the same meal to meal or day to day because it will become all about what you need in the moment to feel satisfied.

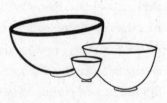

One warning, though: don't trick yourself into thinking you should do things like swap out for a smaller plate. This message tells your brain that you think you aren't worthy or equal to the others around you. Instead of worrying about the size of your plate, follow the method. Serve yourself half and eat as slowly as you can. If you're with others, when you're done, sit back and enjoy their company. If you find that you're eating faster than everyone else, you need to slow down even more. Because this might be uncomfortable, and the brain doesn't like discomfort, you might find it challenging. I get it. But if your goal is to lose weight, and learn how to keep it off, and to have a normal relationship with food, stay in this moment.

You can even look at this like an experiment. Get in the habit of asking yourself, *Why am I having the thought to eat?* and *How hungry am I right now?* Ask yourself why you want that other half. Is it because you don't want to waste it? Did it taste good? Being honest with yourself can be hard because we are pleasure seekers, so it's easy to be seduced by delicious food. But it will still be there when your stomach growls later.

You may be asking, "What do I do with the food on my plate when I feel satisfied midmeal?" To which I answer: "leftovers!" (I am the president of the Leftovers Fan Club. I have enough Tupperware for each individual noodle to have its own personal container.) You can always eat that delicious spaghetti the next time your stomach asks for it.

And I get it, sometimes food spoils quickly. But you are not a trash can. Your body is not a landfill. Any food that your body doesn't need is waste; eating it does not give it any purpose. It won't be used for energy—it will just be stored as fat (or, to be frank, pooped out as literal waste). Whether it is going down the garbage chute or into your esophagus, it's not any less wasteful. If you can save it for another meal, great—but if you can't, please don't treat yourself like a trash can. After all, food doesn't make us overweight, overeating food makes us overweight. I know that for many not finishing everything on their plate is a major sore spot, a trigger. This immediately will cause us to flip our lid and rationalize why eating the rest of the food is a good idea. But remember food is fuel, and unless you are still hungry, do not eat more. Do not let your mind bully you. You are in control, and you can have the rest later when you need it.

TAKING ACTION

Write down some of your fears about starting with a half portion. Can you find a way to see it differently? A curious mind leads us to trust this moment and our thoughts change. Fear makes us narrow-minded. The thing we fear becomes the only thought we have.

"Half won't be enough; I am afraid I will still be hungry." Replace that with *Maybe it will be enough. I can have more in fifteen minutes if I am still hungry.*

"I'm going to miss out on yummy food." Replace that with *I can save some for later or eat this same meal tomorrow.*

Feel free to share your own fears:

_____

_____

Now replace that fear-based thought with the truth: *I can have more if I am hungry soon. It's not going anywhere. I am okay.*

THE RULE #1
WRAP-UP

Eat When You're Hungry

Get your bearings so you can better understand your body and the sensation of physical hunger, which is a sensation in your stomach. It's not scary, and it doesn't affect your energy. If you find it difficult at first, keep asking yourself, *Am I hungry? How do I know? Is this feeling of hunger in my stomach?*

Rate Your Hunger

Use the hunger scale (see page 51) to record your level of hunger before you eat and your satiety level after you eat. It doesn't matter what time of day it is, how many meals you've had that day, and who else is or isn't eating—if you aren't hungry, don't eat! If you are hungry, eat, and start with half. Do not be afraid to close the kitchen after dinner. There will be more food tomorrow.

Identify Your Triggers

Take the time to better understand the triggers that can cause you to slip into your irrational mind. Do your best to avoid those situations whenever possible, and recognize nobody can stop themselves from being triggered. It's inevitable, so when it happens, assure yourself that it's only temporary. Identify emotional eating and cravings for what they truly are, and don't indulge or give in to temptation.

Practice Recognizing Your Cravings

Just try it. You now know the difference between hunger and a craving. Identify those cravings for what they are and ride them out for five days. Remind yourself that you are conducting an experiment. It's temporary. In five days, you can have all the candy, junk food, or whatever else you may be craving that you desire. Try it and see what happens. Following through will give you the strength to better control your reactions in the future.

Apply the Fifteen-Minute Trick

When you do eat, start with half of your normal portion and wait fifteen minutes. Don't let fear consume you. Instead of giving in to your irrational mind, use your rational mind to convince yourself that you will not starve. Know that there will always be more food. Keep practicing your progress and trust yourself, and you will begin to change your abusive relationship with food.

Be Flexible with Your Normal Portion

People love structure, which is why they love a new shiny diet. We cannot predict every moment of every day. We eat at home, at the office, on vacations, in foreign countries, while stressed, while moving through life, and on the go. But everywhere you eat, eat only when you are hungry, take your normal portion, and cut it in half. Beyond that, be flexible in how, what, and where you eat. Adapt to how much you need from day to day and from moment to moment.

Don't be concerned with perfection—it will get easier the more you practice. Keep your focus on progress over perfection. If you aren't used to paying attention to your body this way, it might take a little while for these habits to stick, but have patience with yourself. After some time, you may even know when one bite of food will be too much (trust me, I know clients who can now pinpoint it that accurately). Just keep in mind that health isn't about one decision. It's really hundreds of smaller decisions, small wins that pave the way and add up to determine our overall quality of life. And lastly, please remember you are not a trash can.

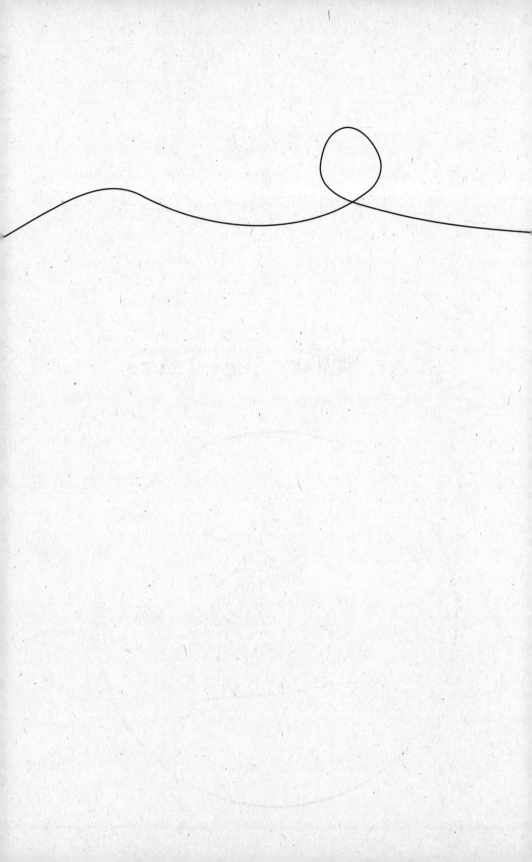

RULE #2

EAT WHAT YOU LOVE

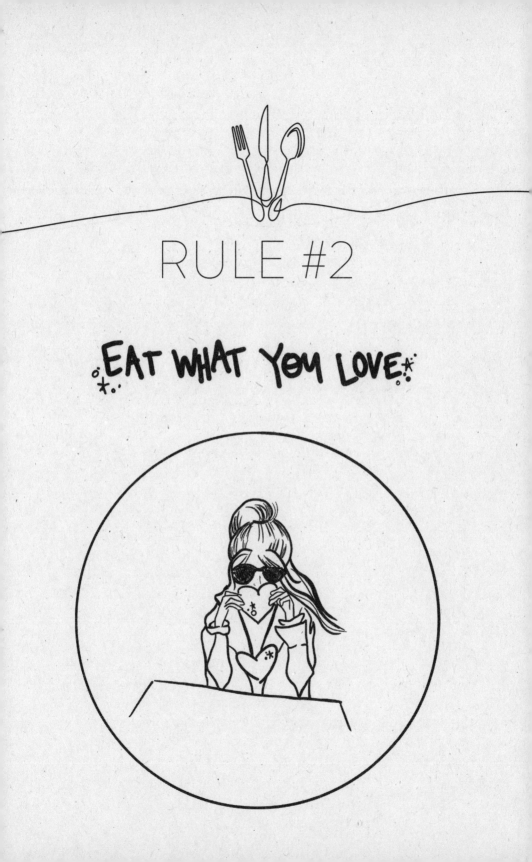

✳ 4 ✳

EAT WHAT YOU LOVE—LUCKY CHARMS
FOR BREAKFAST, LUNCH, AND DINNER

Now we know *when* to eat, so let's talk about *what* to eat . . . You ready? Eat . . . whatever you want.

I get a lot of funny looks from clients when they reach this rule. As former habitual dieters, they've become accustomed to being told what they're supposed to eat. The weird trends people bring to me are endless: "Don't eat after 5 PM," "Only eat celery," "Carrots are high in sugar," "Use this new exotic superfood in every other meal."

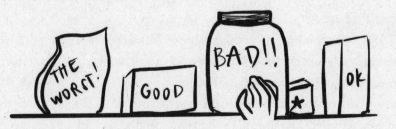

They're so programmed to follow instructions that when I ask them what they like to eat, they're stumped! A lot of people don't remember what their favorite food tastes like because it has been covered in barbed wire and BEWARE signs for years. We make donuts and candy the dangerous, bad-boy, heartthrob that consumes our thoughts. We know Mr. Cake Pop isn't good for us, but he makes us feel so alive! So, after months of avoiding the junk food aisle, we lose the battle. We binge. We overeat. We've given the scary, "unhealthy" foods so much power that we lose control of our decision-making when they're around. Enough!

This rule often causes people to tense up and become fearful because they interpret "eat what you love" as encouragement to binge. That's not what I'm saying. Eating what you love is not permission to eat more than you need. You still must follow Rule #1 and only eat when you are hungry (and still start with half!), or this rule won't work.

But you can absolutely eat the bread, and you can eat the candy! We aren't dieting. You don't want to restrict yourself. There is absolutely no reason that you can't sustain your weight loss (or even avoid gaining weight in the first place) while still enjoying alcohol, ice cream, bread, candy, and all the foods you love. In fact, I promise that you can eat what you want and still lose weight— when we heal our relationship with food, we are no longer controlled by temptations or cravings. Food takes its place as only one important part of our life, as nourishment.

Look, you may be one of the people for whom this rule creates so much freedom that you don't know what to do. This is especially true if you have spent a great deal of time following other people's diets and eating what you think you "should" be eating.

Don't overthink it. Keep things simple. When you're stuck or are feeling overwhelmed, just eat what you love—when you are hungry. Start there. If you are hungry in your stomach, then there is room to eat. Your body doesn't know what you are eating. Stop telling yourself it does. Do you know that if you are overweight and have high cholesterol, and/or high blood pressure, and/ or high blood sugars, and/or high triglycerides and you lose weight, these levels go down as well—no matter what food you ate while losing that weight? Of course, these levels might lower more quickly if we change the types of food we eat. But that does not result in sustainable results.

By eating when you are hungry and starting with half, you will lose weight. By eating what you love and removing any labels around food, you will put yourself on a path of discovering what is right for you. And if you think you are hungry and you find yourself unsure whether or not you want ice cream or a turkey burger, then do not eat. You might be caught in a mindless emotional act, and you aren't hungry. As we discussed earlier, hunger only goes away with food; emotions that cause the thoughts that food is a good idea pass when we put off eating. I need you to practice putting space between the thought to eat and the action to eat.

TAKING ACTION

Forget about what you should eat. Take away the "should" and you take away the guilt. Instead, think about what you "could" and "will" eat when you are hungry. Make a list of foods you love. Or think you love. And write down why you haven't allowed yourself to eat them. Then drop the label you've attached. An example of a label might be: healthy, unhealthy, good, bad, should, shouldn't. Let food be food.

I'm giving you permission and the freedom to eat what you love. We all know that kale is healthy—I don't need to tell you that. I've lost count of the number of clients who have said to me, "I know exactly what's healthy, but I still don't eat it." That is why I'm not going to tell you what foods to eat. You can eat whatever you want. Eating healthy food doesn't lead to sustainable weight loss and maintenance if your relationship with food isn't working.

Yes, I'm giving you permission to eat Lucky Charms for breakfast, lunch, and dinner! And guess what, you will still lose weight while doing it. But when you're choosing what to eat, think back to what we discussed in Rule #1: why you eat. Our childhood experiences may tell us food is a solution for problems that have nothing to do with a hollow feeling in our belly. Do you eat to entertain yourself when you're bored or to calm your anxiety? Does food cheer you up when you're down? What complicated emotional expectations do you have for that poor piece of bread?

I want you to stop worrying about the "healthiest" foods according to your best friend with the killer bod or the latest YouTube beauty guru. Throw out the word altogether. Instead, listen to your body. How do you feel after you eat a bag of chips? Are you satisfied? Do you have the energy you need to get through the next few hours until your next meal? If not, consider a different food next time. Make decisions about what you eat based on self-love and trust, not based on fears put on you by outside influences.

Tiffany was twelve and overweight. Her parents took her to her favorite diner every Friday night, and every week she asked for a milkshake. "You can have it after you finish your burger and fries," her mom would say—which was exactly the problem.

I told her parents to let her have the shake. It took them a couple of weeks before they trusted me and this process enough to just let Tiffany have the milkshake—but then after a few weeks of only eating the shake, she stopped wanting it. For a child who was constantly being told no, being able to have the freedom to choose was a game changer. And, as expected, she said it wasn't satisfying. For Tiffany and her family this lesson was huge. She never ordered the shake again. Imagine if you stopped limiting, restricting, denying yourself foods you love. This would actually give you a chance to see if the love was real or a fantasy.

You can try something similar: the next time you go out to eat, eat what you love, start with half, and wait fifteen minutes to see if you need more food. What did you discover? Do it every time you eat. And once you stop limiting, restricting, and denying yourself, you won't want as much. You will be more satisfied. How many times have you really wanted a burger only to eat the salad and then go home and eat more because you were not satisfied? We can stop doing that. Change is in the air.

I get how strange this sounds. I went to grad school in the SnackWell's era when everyone was afraid of fat. Today, fat isn't the issue, but people are terrified of gluten and bread. Some people just have it in their heads that they can't eat carbs. For a long time, we've all been taught that there are correct things to eat. But no matter what you think you can and can't eat, forget everything you think you know about food.

There is no generic right or wrong food right now. Diets have always given you a false sense of security, telling you what foods are the right foods—but what if those foods aren't right for *you*?

The relationship you have with food is a connection that only you can have. To heal your relationship, you have to go back to the beginning. For this connection to be healthy, the focus needs to be on what you have, not what you don't have. It needs to be flexible. Food is delicious—or, at least, the food I love is delicious to me. I don't have to love your food. You do. And your food should be delicious to you. Food should not be a source of shame, regret, or pain. We have friends telling us what is "off-limits" or counting macros, and these same friends telling us that they are going to be "bad" tonight because they are out for dinner. From this point on, your focus with food is to eat it because you love it, not because your waiter suggested it. You don't even know this waiter. But you do know yourself, and if you don't, this is your opportunity to get to know yourself.

From a weight perspective, your body doesn't know what you are eating. A calorie is a calorie is a calorie. Food is pasta, cake, smoothies, vegetables, steak, and tuna noodle casserole. The body reacts and will absorb every single nutrient you ingest, whether from ice cream or strawberries. Our bodies are sponges that absorb everything, so it doesn't matter if the food is "healthy" or not. Your body doesn't judge you. That's your mind judging you, and it can be overwhelming at times, but it doesn't have to be that way.

DON'T TRY; ALLOW

Consider how you feel about "trying" something. This may evoke feelings of restriction; your chest might feel tight; and you might be bracing yourself for impact. Trying implies that we might not succeed, which can be really scary. So how do you feel about "allowing" something instead? Allowing may feel more open, under your control, something you can prepare for or at least flow with even if you aren't prepared. Can you allow yourself to be in each moment, trusting you are capable of handling the moment with everything you have inside of you rather than needing an external source to help you cope?

What is temptation? Simply put, "it's the desire to do something, especially something wrong or unwise."[1] I teach my clients to see temptation. I teach them that temptations are everywhere and that we are constantly being tested to see how much we have grown, learned, changed. If you are running because you "have to" get in shape but hate running, you likely won't keep it up. The temptation to skip a day is strong. If you are on a restricted food plan and go to a party where they are serving your favorite little cheese things, the temptation to eat it is overwhelming. If you don't eat dairy but are traveling to Europe, the temptation to eat gelato every day is all consuming. Temptation is everywhere.

Okay, so what? Here is what you need to know. In a study on self-control, the researchers found that "the people who said they excelled at self-control were hardly using it at all."[2] And furthermore, in a later study researchers found "that students who exerted more self-control were not more successful in accomplishing their goals. It was the students who experienced fewer temptations overall who were more successful."[3] What this means for you is that if you intentionally create a routine and have fun while you do it, then it won't feel like you are exerting self-control because those fun routines will help you avoid temptation. It will be easier to pursue goals because they will feel more effortless. In the past, your goal was short term: lose weight. Now your goal is to be well and balanced, to have peace of mind around food and your health, and to have a healthy relationship with food. You need to engage in activities that don't feel like a chore.

There are some really good dieters out there—you all know them. But those great dieters see everything as being either black or white—all or none, good or bad. To have a healthy, sustainable relationship with food, though, I don't want you to be too disciplined. I would rather you be curious. Don't sensationalize diet plans. There are no prizes for being a good dieter, because diets end, and life goes on.

Don't get me wrong. If you cut out certain foods, stick to a diet plan, and eat what's healthy, you will lose weight. I'm not disputing that. The problem is that you won't be able to keep it off because you didn't lose it under the right circumstances, and you aren't eating what you love. Eventually, that disciplined dieter who forces herself to eat salad when she hates it will reach her breaking point.

Other researchers found that "People who are good at self-control . . . seem to be structuring their lives in a way to avoid having to make a self-control decision in the first place."[4] That's why each of my rules gives you structure instead of being about willpower. In my experience, people who repeat the same activities, such as scheduled exercise, walks, or meditation, have an easier time fulfilling their goals because they've planned ahead. And these accomplishments create feelings of pride, strength, and inner power.

When it comes to changing your relationship with food, losing weight, keeping it off, and improving your health, it is a matter of allowing yourself to stay in flow without restriction. If you feel restricted, stop and evaluate what is happening. Your aim is the ability to develop habits and to be consistent. Inner power is what says, "a cookie won't solve my problems," or "buying another purse won't make me feel any better," or "a drink isn't going to make my rent cheaper." Someone with inner power says, "Okay, in this moment, it may not be easy, but I have survived every other moment 100 percent of the time. I am ready."

One thing to keep in mind, though: eat the cookie not just because you want to, but because you are hungry and it's what you love. Don't eat it just because you're tempted to. Things like cheat days are temptations, and they are no longer necessary, because any time you're hungry, you eat what you love.

Of course, you can love something and not desire it. You can also desire something and not love it for your body. Think about being on the beach right now—maybe this sounds like a great idea, but it doesn't mean you need to get to the beach right now. We can coexist with this desire without acting on it. Just because you love a cookie doesn't mean you need to eat a cookie every time you remember that you love cookies.

The sky is beautiful in that there is a constant stream of colors and moving clouds. Sometimes the sky is clear. Sometimes clouds bring storms that are small and quick, while others last much longer. You build inner power by showing up every day, rain or shine, and learning to stay in the discomfort while gaining trust in yourself. This requires balancing your backpack on the journey, constantly staying connected to the spokes on your Wellness Wheel, being open to learning, and making sure your self-care matches what your body is trying to tell you.

That power is refined by making every meal about nourishing your body and seeing the difference between eating for hunger and eating for comfort. It's about having the freedom to love and enjoy what you eat, not trying to see how long you can keep eating specific foods while not eating others. You do all of that so when the storm does come, your muscle memory kicks in and quickly and efficiently grounds you. Inner power teaches you to never underestimate your control because this control is now a source of fun and pride as opposed to willpower, which is temporary.

In the end, it all goes back to knowing your *why*.

As we move further in understanding Rule #2, I want to help you change your focus from how this may feel hard in the beginning to the big picture, the long-term goal. Without knowing your *why*, it's harder to convince yourself that you're doing something positive for your long-term health, and it's easier to think that you're missing out on something that you used to love. Once you start feeling like that, old habits creep back in.

This doesn't mean that you have to continually ask yourself why in every moment, and your *why* doesn't have to be some gargantuan goal—no matter how big you may have made it earlier in this book. Sometimes the *why* is as simple as feeling good and balanced throughout the day. Your mind just has to be in the moment. Staying present is the key to using your *why*. As you practice seeing temptations as mere temptations, you will need to remember to use the new skill of finding your mind when it gets excited over things like the just-delivered chocolate iced blended coffee drink that was sent to you as a thank-you. This coffee wasn't your idea and just because it's in front of you does not mean you need to drink it. You can save it for later if you love it, for when you get hungry, or you can regift it and take full ownership of the thoughtfulness of the sender.

"I'm having that later" translates in your body to "no one is taking my food away." These positive thoughts actually fill you with gusto to carry on, making what was once a chore something fun and aligned with your goal. When living through uncertain times, your self-care is still a priority. Eating what you love is standing up for your body. Speak your truth. Eat what you love. Be your biggest advocate. At the end of the day, you will be thinking, *I've got this*, rather than *I will try again tomorrow.* Inner power is staying power that will require you to retrain your mind.

TAKING ACTION

A person with inner power is a person who has the strength to show up every day and take care of themselves, who is postured in the moment to put the needs of their body, heart, and emotional well-being first. Now this person is learning to use that same strength in the moments of discomfort to instead align with their *why*.

Repeat ten times: "I have everything I need inside of me to survive this moment."

✳ 5 ✳

EAT WHAT YOU LOVE—
THE SCIENCE-Y PART

When I first started my practice, I provided every client with a thorough break-down on every single nutrient and how it affected the body. I didn't get far into my spiel before I'd see their eyes glaze over. Some even yawned, and I don't blame them. Nutrition and digestion are compli-cated and can be boring. But I still have to explain how the body processes food, because it's so much easier to develop an approach to eating when you understand 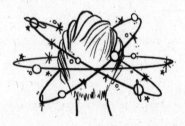 what's happening inside the body and why—and trust me when I say the way our bodies can efficiently take in everything we give it and use it to heal us (or, sadly, harm us) is actually awesome.

Here's the CliffsNotes version: the digestive tract is one long slinky that runs from your mouth to your anus. (I'm sure your seven-year-old self is crack-ing up at that word—you're welcome—but stick with me.) If untangled and stretched out, that tube is thirty feet long, and every single inch of it has a job. Essentially, everything you eat is digested (broken down), and then absorbed in this tract. Everything moves down and through your digestive tract. A healthy gut or digestive tract needs to be able to break down, absorb, and store the magic inside the food.

For the purpose of this explanation, let's say that you are an average, healthy individual, and your body runs efficiently. Starting from the beginning, you see and smell food, which initiates the making of saliva and alerts your stomach food is coming in. When you chew your food, enzymes in your saliva get to work breaking it down. Chewing is the only mechanical breakdown of food we'll get, so do it well. One study in the *American Journal of Clinical Nutrition* asked the participants to chew each bite forty times and found that when participants chewed their food a little more than usual, they ate less, and their gut hormones related to hunger, and satiety improved.[1] Chewing well helps prevent digestive disorders. Not to mention the faster you eat, the more food you tend to eat. Slowing your pace and chewing more can reduce your overall food intake.[2]

When we swallow, a flap called the epiglottis covers the lungs, so we don't choke and the food can travel down to the esophagus. Next, the walls of the esophagus create contractions that keep the food moving downward. There are sphincters at the top and the bottom of the esophagus that act as a clog to keep our food from coming back up or going down too fast. When you experience heartburn, the acid from your stomach (which is supposed to be there) gets through the lower sphincter (into the esophagus, where it's very definitely not supposed to be). We call it reflux, and it's related to a ton of digestive disorders, but it's fixable.[3]

Your stomach serves a few purposes. First, to store food (about four cups or one liter) where it will be slowly digested over a four- to six-hour window. Second, it acts like a nest, so the acid rakes over everything in the stomach to kill any harmful viruses, bacteria, or fungus.[4] As food mixes with the acids, it's ready to continue its journey. The stomach also uses contractions to mix your food with acids and enzymes to further break it down, or digest it. Your stomach is lined with a mucosal layer to prevent the acid from causing you any harm, but if that mucosal layer gets damaged, you will feel it. Your food is now considered chyme, a thick liquid.

Now let's meet the duodenum (ten inches long), jejunum (eight feet long), and ileum (twelve feet long), which make up what is otherwise known as the small intestine. This is where 90 percent of digestion and absorption occur. At this point, your body leans on chemicals (acid, bile, and enzymes) to further break down those nutrients. Contractions still move the bolus (food) through the tract. The nutrients from your food, while still in your intestines, have now been made small enough to cross through the walls (epithelial layer) from your intestine to your bloodstream.[5] Do you remember learning about diffusion, osmosis, and active transport back in science class? It's okay if you don't, but that's what's basically happening inside of you—and it happens automatically . . . we hope. The transfer of nutrients (our lifeline) from our digestive tract to our bloodstream (our bloodstream carries the nutrients to the necessary cells for use or storage) can unfortunately have a few hiccups. Sometimes unchewed or large food particles can cross over, sometimes our microbiome is lacking and our defense system is down, and sometimes high levels of stress and high levels of cortisol decrease our gut barrier.[6] There are many reasons why we can have a kink in the system, and my best advice would be to love your body and listen when it's sending you messages, take a deep breath before you eat, and eat when you are hungry.

The large intestine is about six feet long and made up of four parts: ascending colon, transverse colon, descending colon, and the sigmoid colon. At this point, food has been in your digestive tract for about six to eight hours. Your food, chyme, is now prepped and ready to absorb any remaining water and salts (sodium, potassium, electrolytes, and so on), while eliminating any leftovers (bacteria or waste) to form stool.[7] The poop hardens because it's been dehydrated. It is now ready to sit and wait in your rectum. The anal sphincter is the only thing holding it in. (I can hear your seven-year-old self laughing again!)

The liver is another important organ we should discuss. The many jobs of the liver include metabolizing fats, proteins, and carbohydrates; excreting cholesterol, hormones, and drugs; storing glycogen, vitamins, and minerals; and detoxifying and purifying your blood.[8] Think of your liver as your bodyguard.

It's responsible for circulating blood sugar to keep you fueled and functioning. It also stores blood sugar in the form of glucose.

The glucostatic theory compares the liver to a gas tank that constantly monitors if we are empty or full of blood sugar, and I've seen how beneficial this theory can be for weight loss and weight maintenance.[9] The theory claims that low blood sugar initiates a need for food and drives our behavior to eat. This is specifically why I tell you to eat every two to three hours, and to be hungry when you eat. Regulating your blood sugar is the most important part of signaling to your body that you are safe. Low blood sugar is also linked to a significant increase in overeating, which causes weight gain and glucose intolerance. And some data even suggests this increase in fat gain is our body's amazing way of protecting us from starvation.[10]

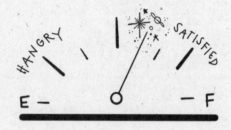

Now let me introduce you to three specific hormones: ghrelin, leptin, and insulin. These are the hormones behind the scenes, the ones telling your mind when to eat and how much to eat.

Ghrelin is secreted from the lining of an empty stomach and travels to your brain to say, "Hey, I'm hungry." That's when you feel hunger pangs. Ghrelin levels will keep rising until you eat, and ignoring them will eventually lead to a primal level that fuels out-of-control eating.

Leptin is made in your fat tissues when it's time to eat. It also sends signals to your brain (hypothalamus) to signal that you're satisfied or full. We need to slow down the rate at which we eat to give this hormone a chance to say, "Hey, you have had enough for now."

Insulin regulates blood sugar. If you wait too long to eat, you might feel hungry, shaky, and weak because your blood sugar levels have dropped. That's when your body needs carbohydrates, which are broken down with help from your saliva. These carbs are fuel. They become blood sugar, or gasoline for the engine that is our body.

These hormones control how your body feels. Here is a list of common outside factors that can affect those hormones, and ultimately how you feel:

+ lack of sleep
+ too much sleep
+ stress
+ processed foods
+ lack of exercise
+ too much exercise
+ environmental toxins
+ chemicals
+ lack of socializing
+ staring at your phone or computer screen at night

This book and the habits you are creating will help by putting you in balance, allowing these hormones in your body to instruct and guide you.

YOUR METABOLISM

Our bodies are designed to be efficient metabolic machines. Your metabolism is constantly providing your body with energy (calories or fuel) for every basic function such as breathing, sleeping, thinking, and digesting. It's dependent on your sex, age, weight, height, physical exercise, and medications.

If you think you have a slow metabolism (and your doctor says it's not your thyroid—and by the way, it's unlikely for it to be your thyroid), then there is a very good chance it's your current diet, diet history, and your body fat percentage. But it doesn't matter if your metabolism is fast or slow; you can change it in a matter of days just by getting and staying consistent.

Picture a stove with six burners. If you have a slow metabolism, you might only have two of these burners on. The rest are off. Imagine having to cook Thanksgiving dinner on a stove with only two burners. That would take days. Our goal is to turn all six on and to *keep* them on. That is what eating every two to three hours (and moving your body—we'll get more into that later) does. We maintain a low burn in our metabolism by eating consistently enough that the burners flow naturally instead of slowing down—or worse, turning off. A low burn means the body is efficient, and when that happens maintaining weight is easy-peasy. (That's why I call hunger your best friend—it's a sign that your metabolism is kicking. If you didn't get hungry, that would mean you have a very slow metabolism and you would be overeating all of the time. That's how you gain weight.)

TAKING ACTION

Do you wear a fitness tracker or bracelet or anything else on your wrist? If so, here is what I want you to do: each and every time you have a single thought about food, I want you to take off your watch or bracelet and switch wrists. The goal is for you to recognize that you can eat anything you love, *when* you are hungry. This exercise will help you retrain your mind. It will also help put space between the thought to eat and the action to eat. After a few rounds of this, you will begin to notice how mindlessly we often act. This practice will empower you—and that is what we need more of.

Some examples of thoughts you might have that can inspire an accessory change: *Should I eat that? Can I eat that? Is this healthy? How many calories are in this? When was the last time I ate? Will this food make me feel sick? Why am I eating this? . . .*

✳ 6 ✳

EAT WHAT YOU LOVE—UNLESS IT'S
MAKING YOU SICK

There is one caveat to eating what you love, and you'll thank me for it: the foods you love cannot make you sick. What do I mean by sick? How many times have you felt any one of the following symptoms?

- ✦ congestion
- ✦ gas
- ✦ bloating
- ✦ diarrhea
- ✦ constipation
- ✦ headache
- ✦ heartburn
- ✦ runny nose
- ✦ rashes
- ✦ joint pain
- ✦ fatigue

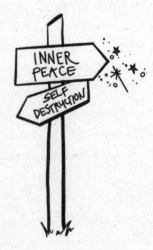

✦ grogginess
✦ sleeplessness

I could keep going with this list, but you get the idea. For some people, these symptoms can be major problems that change the way you live your life, or they might be minor inconveniences—but either way, it's not okay to feel any of these things. It's not normal! In fact, it's a sign that your digestive tract isn't balanced. The foods you are eating could be causing these symptoms. Most of these ailments wouldn't bring us to the doctor, but they should. They are signs that your body needs some extra support and attention.

It could be that every time you eat a banana, you get heartburn, but bananas are "good" for you, so you keep eating them. Or you feel like taking a nap after every meal—and why do you get an upset stomach from eating oatmeal when there isn't even gluten in it? It's because what's healthy for me is not what is healthy for you. Blueberries are a food loaded with antioxidants that might be really good for you, but they make me sick. Healthy is a label that we are going to stop using—at least until we understand that we are not the same.

Another reason why one-size-fits-all diets don't work is because foods affect people differently. One food that your friend loves and relies on to lose weight could cause you to be bloated. Your body is different from everyone else's because we live different lives, and our bodies have had different experiences. Those experiences may include allergies, stress, medications, antibiotics, trauma, childhoods, cultural differences in our diets, vitamins, vaccines, and so on. To permanently fix our relationship with food, we need to be in our own bodies and stop comparing.

You've likely heard a lot about "superfoods," and you've certainly heard about foods that are "bad" for you, but do you really know which foods are making *you* sick? Once you know that, you have the power to see the magic in food.

Back in the day, I used to call myself a food detective because I was able to root out everyone's food sensitivity issue. And I was good! Ten years ago, I had a client from New Orleans in his fifties who had already gone through both of his kidneys and was now waiting to get another transplant. The first thing I did was learn more about his background and diet. If you've studied epidemiology, you understand that when you grow up in different parts of the country, and in different cultures, you likely grew up eating different foods and making different lifestyle choices. That makes you susceptible to different digestive conditions because of those foods and behaviors.

Once he told me what he was eating, I recognized that those foods were high in oxalic acid. In a case like his, health professionals often assume that calcium stones were the problem, but they rarely consider oxalic acid, which is found in rhubarb pie, tea, berries, wine, and chocolate. Once we were able to change his diet, his kidney function improved. When his doctor at Stanford called me, I thought he was going to be upset. Instead, he was shocked by how I saved him from having to undergo another kidney transplant. I'd love to take a victory lap, but any registered dietitian would be able to recognize what was going on given the client's background and diet. The problem is that it's not a question that everyone asks.

Question: So how do you figure out which foods are causing you harm?

Answer: Start with a simple process of elimination. If you came to me and said you were experiencing any physical symptoms (your body's alert system) after breakfast when you ate yogurt, blueberries, and cashew milk, the first thing we'd need to figure out is the underlying cause of your symptoms. We'd also look at your family history. We know that our DNA matters, but so does our lifestyle. For instance, if you have a family history of high cholesterol, does this mean you'll have it as well?

Sugars from carbs, like the lactose from yogurt, will affect you within fifteen minutes after eating, while proteins don't affect you for two to four hours. So the next day, I'd say try yogurt and blueberries, but leave out the cashew milk and see how you feel. If that didn't fix anything, keep switching out each ingredient one at a time, and go through the process of elimination with each ingredient. Eventually, you will pinpoint the food that gives you digestive issues.

The problem is that life is not always this simple. Rarely do people eat the same thing two days in a row, and the number of times the average person eats out and orders take-out food further complicates things. That makes it difficult to pinpoint the specific ingredient that could be causing digestive issues, especially since most people have more than one sensitivity. However, a good place to start is ruling out what is not giving you issues, because too many people make the mistake of assuming or misdiagnosing themselves.

EVERYTHING, EVERYTHING IS AFFECTED BY THE BACTERIA IN THE HUMAN BODY

Bacteria are everywhere in and on our body: on our skin, up our nose, in our gut—and they provide very important functions that are essential to our well-being, health, and survival. These bacteria are part of our microbiome. Here are just a few roles bacteria play: they control how we store fat and how we break down nutrients; they replace damaged cells with new ones (which is vital in preventing disease); they affect how we smell; and they regulate and influence our brain through hormones. The good news is that our diet plays a huge role in maintaining this harmonic balance of bacteria in our body. The bad news is that sometimes we are out of balance and that affects the way we digest our food. Food that quite possibly had never been an issue before, and is possibly food you love, might become toxic to your body now.

The food we eat has millions of microbes in every bite. Changing the type of food we eat, from meat to beans, can affect the type of microbes we let into our body. These little bacteria change and multiply quickly; they evolve and adapt and make up about 1 to 3 percent of our body's mass; and what's more, they outnumber our human cells by ten to one.[1] Knowing our microbiome system exists and thinking of it as an organ that plays a huge role in your health will help you understand why you may experience some changes in the way food makes you feel. Even food you love.

IT ALL CONNECTS TO THE GUT

Food is the beginning, middle, and end of your health, but on your journey, you might have been misled, or slipped up, and unintentionally harmed your digestive system, leaving you unwell. If your gut is not healthy, you aren't absorbing and digesting that food properly. Besides for digesting and absorbing things, you also need a healthy gut to provide a barrier to prevent harmful agents crossing your bloodstream. When I say "gut," I'm talking about your stomach and intestine. Think of it like a hose. It's thick and there are multiple layers, but we're only going to talk about three parts:

+ The mucosal layer: the inner layer of your hose
+ Tight junctions: a fence that seals the mucosal and epithelium layers
+ The epithelium layer: the outer layer of your hose

The mucosal layer is the gut's first line of defense. If that's weakened, the contents of the gut can leak through the inner layers of your intestinal wall, and potentially into your bloodstream, which opens the floodgates to potential disease. There are multiple factors that contribute to this inflammatory issue known as "leaky gut." The loss of our intestinal barrier can occur suddenly after injecting various poisons, leading to major trauma and full body sepsis, but it can also occur slowly over time. Here are some factors that can lead to a reduction of your defenses:

+ Small intestinal bacterial overgrowth (SIBO): a condition where there is an imbalance or excess of small intestinal bacteria. Some common symptoms of SIBO include bloating, gas, distension, and diarrhea.[2]
+ Small intestinal fungal overgrowth (SIFO): a recent study found that an "overgrowth of fungus in the gastrointestinal tract might be the root cause for more than 25% of IBS (irritable bowel syndrome) patients."[3]
+ Parasites and/or foodborne illnesses can cause long-term or short-term imbalances in our microflora that create significant nutritional deficiencies and hormone disturbances that can then affect our memory, our mood, our digestion, and our immune response.[4]
+ Psychological stress, sleep deprivation, environmental conditions (high altitude, heat, and cold), pollutants, physical stress (exercising too much or too little), and diet (too much food, too little food, and poor food choices) all affect the gut microbiome, thus affecting the way we respond to any of the above.
+ Antibiotics, medications, and chronic use of painkillers disrupt the gut microbiome. Gut health requires the proper balance of bacteria. Diversity of our microbiome is essential and, unfortunately, some

common medications that kill bad bacteria are also killing our good bacteria. It is necessary to address this challenge and to have a strategy in place that includes probiotics.

✦ Chronic use of antacids: proton pump inhibitors are meant to lower stomach acid to prevent heartburn or gastroesophageal reflux disease (GERD); they are important but meant to be used short term. Avoiding them would be super, but understanding the root cause of your digestive discomfort is a better route if possible.

✦ Age: as we get older, our gut microbiome changes.

Normally, our gut functions at the highest level, and we never notice any issues. A healthy person can recover from a stomach bug in twenty-four hours because the body responds by turning the immune response on. Think of that immune response like a sneeze, or your body's way of rejecting something. But when the body is overtaxed, and that mucosal layer is repeatedly weakened, it becomes much harder to turn that immune response off—and some people can't at all. It gets stuck in the "on" position, creating an autoimmune response as your body works overtime to get back to a balanced state. That's a big problem. In addition to added inflammation and digestive issues like irritable bowel syndrome, a poor diet, unhealthy lifestyle, added stress, and certain medications can lead to almost all disease states.

When you eat foods that make you sick, it's your body's way of screaming at you and letting you know that the lining of your gut has been damaged. Remember that this is your journey, and not all foods work for everyone.

Get curious about what works for you, because sometimes these digestive issues are the first sign that we have a bigger problem brewing. You can talk to your doctor or a dietitian about finding a test to help you know what foods are triggering your gut and making you feel sick. The good news is that you are in control of how well your digestive tract works.

THE TRUTH ABOUT FOOD INTOLERANCE

Everyone thinks they're sensitive to gluten. Everyone! Maybe not everyone, but many people assume that every digestive condition they experience is because of an intolerance to gluten. (I do want to point out that we are discussing food intolerances or sensitivities; we are not discussing allergies. Allergies don't really go away and can get worse over time; sensitivities are temporary.) Back in graduate school, I learned that there is a very small percentage of people who are allergic to gluten, so I'm quick to assume that the issues my clients describe are likely of another nature. Gluten intolerance will show up in a blood test, but there are certain symptoms that do indicate a particular food intolerance.

Jessica is a client of mine who is in her sixties now. When she was seventeen, a doctor told her that she had irritable bowel syndrome, and that it was a terrible disease that she had to live with. After listening to her symptoms, I could tell right away that she had multiple things going on with her gut. Given her symptoms of airy gas, smelly gas, heartburn, bloating, diarrhea, and constipation, we decided to look into food sensitivities. And we discovered that she had a lot of them. After identifying the problem, we altered her diet and gave her supplemental support so she could begin to heal.

You are in control of your own health. Aside from a serious condition like Crohn's disease or colitis, the most common digestive issues may be a result of taking too many antibiotics, protonics (heartburn, gas, and GERD medicine), eating a poor diet, and being so stressed out that it affects the lining of your gut. Most of these issues you can improve on your own with a little diet and stress support, but there are some great resources out there to better help you identify your true food sensitivities.

When I used to go to the mall with my daughter, she would always ask for a soft pretzel as a snack. I wanted her to connect to her own body without my influence, so I got her a pretzel when asked. It wasn't long before she started to recognize she always got a stomachache soon after eating the pretzel. When she was beginning to see that there was a connection between her stomachaches and the pretzel, I suggested the pretzel could be the cause, and she should try to eat half of what she normally ate and see if she still got a tummy ache. So that is what she did; she ate less and waited. She found that the pretzel still made her feel sick. Once she was able to recognize that, it was easy for her to pick a different snack. I asked her to start with half because telling her "I think the pretzel is making you sick—stop eating it" would have felt like I was taking away her favorite blankie. Instead, I put the ball in her court. And now when she chooses to eat it or not, she is making that decision from a confident mindset rather than a sad, deprived mindset.

I love coffee. I drink coffee every day. There are some days when it feels like I need more than my usual amount of coffee and other days when I don't feel like I need it at all. I remember at one point I was super anxious and drinking coffee made me feel jittery, panicky, and a little sick. This was definitely unusual for me. I wasn't very happy about this particular discovery since I love coffee. One morning, I was about to take my vitamins with my morning coffee and remembered that feeling, so I did a little mental ping-pong with myself and chose water. Thankfully that was short lived and I can have coffee again, but it's a good reminder to be flexible in what we need—that just because we had it yesterday doesn't mean we need it today. Self-care is different for everyone. Don't underestimate the power of knowing how you want to feel (or not feel); knowing that you don't want to feel a certain way can help you make a better decision for your body.

How many times are you willing to burn yourself? Think about it. If you burn your hand when pulling something out of the oven, the next time you'll probably wear an oven mitt. It's the same with food. Once you become more mindful of which foods are making you sick, it becomes easier and more natural to say no to those foods, no matter how much you love(d) them. And just because there is one moment in time when something doesn't agree with you doesn't mean that food is lost forever. I drink coffee almost every morning, but I don't if I'm feeling too wired. The key is to be in the moment and to take care of yourself in the here and now.

If you know that eating bacon will give you a migraine, or celery juice will give you diarrhea, you will have a choice as to whether you want to deal with that. Understanding how certain foods make you feel is what makes Rule #2 so effective. You have permission to eat anything you love when you're hungry, but take note of how it makes you feel after. A food we are sensitive to can affect us after we eat and/or up to three days after. So today you could be experiencing a reaction from something you ate three days ago.

Have you been complaining of feeling imbalanced and not 100 percent? Do you go to the doctor often to find out what might be wrong with you? Sit with that for a while. Really pay attention to how the food you eat makes you feel. You might realize that you've had the answers the whole time. If the ice cream that you're dying to have makes you bloated and sleepy, try eating less and see if you still feel bloated or ready for bed. If this is the case, then you are sensitive to the ice cream or something in the ice cream. But if you try eating less and you don't get bloated or tired, there is a very good chance you were eating more than you needed or more quickly than you should be, and your body was having to work hard to digest. Keep in mind the ice cream section of the supermarket is lengthy—I bet you could find an alternative.

The true benefit of this part of the rule is combining it with Rule #1, because real hunger will lead to a wiser option. Maybe you don't love cookies after all—you were only dying to have them because you weren't allowed to before, or because you sensationalized cookies and made them a reward. But isn't the real reward being well, and having so much freedom and peace around food that you know you can still have that candy when you want it without anxiety, fear, or guilt?

Don't be afraid to eat what you love, especially since we are hardwired to seek pleasure. This rule might seem scary, but it actually prevents us from over-indulging. We are getting pleasure from choosing the foods we love—and since Rule #1 taught us to trust that there is more later, with Rule #2, you can trust yourself to make the right choice now. Remember my client Tiffany who begged her parents for the milkshake back in chapter four: once she had the choice, she ended up choosing what made her body feel good. When you're really experiencing physical hunger, chances are that you will opt for the food that loves you back. It will make you feel satisfied, and the candy will soon be forgotten.

THE MIRACLE OF MODERN SCIENCE

Luckily, you won't require my investigative services. Technology has advanced to the point that there are food sensitivity test kits you can easily take in your home and mail back to get your results in a week (a test kit that you order and send back with a small blood sample). Now, remember that there are food allergies, and there are food sensitivities. If you have a food allergy, you probably know about it, but most people are unaware of the foods to which they are sensitive. So, if you have any concerns, I would seek out a food sensitivity kit and change your life now. It's simple and super easy.

The test measures your body's reactivity to certain foods. (This is not the same thing as a food allergy test.) This test will tell you which foods are doing damage to your gut and making you feel sick. It puts these foods into four categories: moderate, mild, high, and normal.

Obviously, the foods that fall into your "high" category are the ones you are the most sensitive to. You might have a couple of foods in your "mild" or "moderate" category that you frequently eat and don't even realize are bothering you because the symptoms are so mild.

Many people are in denial when they first see their results because it's common for foods they've eaten their entire lives to show up, which makes it difficult for people to wrap their heads around the fact that those foods have been doing them harm.

Nick was a forty-three-year-old client of mine who had been to every gastroenterologist in his area, but none of them were able to treat his gas, bloating, and constipation. He had been placed on antibiotics for small intestinal bacteria overgrowth (SIBO) but none of it helped. When he took the food sensitivity test, we learned that he was highly sensitive to salmon and chicken, two foods he frequently ate. Just by eliminating those foods, we were able to eliminate his symptoms.

Sometimes it's that simple. It's important to know that the symptoms you're experiencing from a food sensitivity may not always be in your gut even though they are starting in your gut. Sometimes the food we eat affects more than our digestion. In other words, you may not always associate your symptoms with the food you eat. But more likely than not the inflammatory response is coming from the foods to which you are sensitive. Some of these symptoms affect our energy or our brain function.

TAKING ACTION

Circle any symptoms you might be feeling:

✦ Headache

✦ Foggy brain (you can't seem to think clearly)

✦ Fatigue (you are ready for a nap after you eat)

✦ Runny nose (do you carry tissues with you?)

✦ Clearing your throat after you eat

✦ Bloating (your stomach feels expanded and full of air)

✦ Diarrhea

✦ Constipation (pooping hard rabbit pellets or golf balls that don't leave you feeling completely empty)

✦ Psoriasis or eczema

✦ Random joint pain that comes and goes

If you have circled any of these, please consider supporting your gut and discovering to what you are sensitive. These symptoms will go away with some attention and changes.

Stephanie was healthy and in great shape; all of her blood tests were normal. She exercised regularly, never got sick, had no signs of high cholesterol or high blood pressure issues, didn't eat sugar, got plenty of sleep, and meditated. She had a level of health we all aspire to achieve. If anyone knew she was seeing me, they would question her motives, but the problem was that her nose ran all the time and her joints ached. So, naturally, I insisted she do a food sensitivity test, and as expected, her test listed only four foods and they all fell into the "mild" category. However, those four foods were foods she ate almost every day. All she had to do was build up the lining of her gut and cut down (or cut out) those four foods for a few weeks. That's what she did, and guess what? Her nose stopped running and joints no longer ached.

Earlier we discussed how overeating can stretch your stomach, which will create discomfort in your body and could aggravate the surrounding organs like your bladder or bowels. This is not the same discomfort you will get from a food to which you are sensitive. It's important to remember that there is a difference between the foods you're sensitive to and the foods you're overeating. You could, of course, be sensitive to foods you don't even eat, as I learned I was when I took my own food sensitivity test. (Peas and beef were on my list, but I've had an aversion to peas since I was a kid and I rarely eat beef, so that was never a problem for me at all.) But you could also just be overeating something. Please pay attention to what your body is trying to tell you—is your digestive tract screaming at you with bloating and gas and diarrhea, or are you uncomfortable from the amount of food you are eating?

Like many of my clients, I was in denial at first when I saw crab on my sensitivity list, and I thought the test had to be wrong. I rarely ate crab. Well, that's not entirely true. I would eat crab when I'd get sushi, which wasn't often, but enough. Like most people, when I saw the results of the test, I immediately went out and ate crab to see what happened. Sure enough, my stomach started to hurt. What was even more revealing was that my hands hurt. That's when I connected the dots. I had experienced minor aches and pains in my hands for years. It was frustrating, and I never went to see the doctor about it (that's another issue), so I never knew why it was happening. Then, I realized that whenever I ate crab, I would feel an ache in my hands, sometimes for a couple of days. There were times when it was too painful for me to even hold a pen. That opened my eyes. Sensitivity to foods can happen over time or suddenly. We become sensitive when we are unable to break down a certain ingredient. It could be that we stopped producing the enzyme needed to digest it, or we took an antibiotic, or we are experiencing more stress than usual. The good news is that sensitivities to certain foods are temporary, and the sooner you pay attention the sooner it goes away.

Who knows what issues you might be suffering from that you never associated with the foods you eat? That's why finding out what foods you are sensitive to is a game changer, and I recommend that everyone take a food sensitivity test. Remember, we are creating a new foundation and a new belief system. Slowly but surely, whether two weeks or two months later, you will say, "Wow, I haven't taken a Tylenol in a while." Or maybe you'll wake up one day and realize that you forgot to worry. Keep in mind the root of most of our "whys" is peace of mind.

So Can You Never Eat These Foods Again?

Many people, upon learning that they are sensitive to certain foods they love, immediately feel restricted and begin to panic. Discovering food sensitivities might feel like a new rock in your backpack, but please hear me out: this is an opportunity for you to find new foods that you can fall in love with.

1. When you are sensitive to a food, try to stop eating it for thirty days to lower your body's stress reaction. You can do it. That's like the definition of self-care—not being abusive and finding things that are good for you. So use this food sensitivity test as a tool to help heal your body. The good news is there is also another way around it if you can't seem to move past the "I love this food so much." Just eat what you're sensitive to when you are hungry and see what happens to your body. The sensitivity usually strikes two to four hours after you eat a food, but can occur up to three days after you eat it. Truly noticing the results might be the spark you need to take care of yourself. Don't see this as negative; instead, see this as an opportunity to help your body heal. Get curious to promote a more balanced, peaceful relationship with food. The idea is to get your gut health back to 100 percent and then try slowly incorporating these foods back into your diet.

2. Take probiotics. For years, everyone used to say that I loved probiotics so much that I should marry them. It was a running joke, but they weren't entirely wrong. Probiotics are important because they contain beneficial bacteria that support our existing microbiome. Every person has around two to six pounds of microbes that comprise the human microbiome.[5] This is our body's first line of defense when it comes to all things wellness. When we take antibiotics to kill off the bad bacteria, they also kill the healthy bacteria. Over time, you can lose more and more of these microbes, and if you are not supporting the ones you have, then you are going to feel unbalanced. Probiotics are like little tourists that bring messages to our microbiome and strengthen the microbiome's economy. They are transient, but very welcome, and necessary, visitors.

3. Eat yogurt. There are probiotics in yogurt that are very important in gut health and healing your gut. Of course, you can buy a probiotic supplement, but if your body can tolerate yogurt, that is a better way to get probiotics. Not just any yogurt, though. Look for one that has five or more microbes listed in the ingredient list. Also try to eat more organic fruits and vegetables. These foods contain antioxidants that will also repair your gut.

4. Eat more fiber. Chia seeds and flax seeds are good because they contain omegas that strengthen and protect the mucosal layer. You need to up your fiber and omegas to help your transit time (the time it takes for food to move from your mouth to the toilet) and allow your body to detox.

5. Eat foods high in flavonoids such as tea, coffee, berries, grapes, and other fruits and vegetables to help lower inflammation. These flavonoids prevent a buildup of stress from our life and our diets.

6. Learn about the possible pesticides and toxins in your food. Then work to eat less of them or remove them from your diet. What you can start to do is buy organic fruits, vegetables, dairy products, and grains. Beware of the white packet you find at the bottom of the plastic container of certain fruits. Even the plastic itself could contain toxins that leach into the fruit. If those are the only fruits or veggies you have, eating them is better than not eating them, but if you have a choice, choose the one that supports your gut. And since we are talking about fruit, keep in mind this won't be the only fruit you will eat this week. You will have lots of opportunity to make choices. Progress over perfection.

7. Don't forget that stress is also toxic. Stress can damage the mucosal layer and increase the body's immune response. We can't prevent stress but we can work on the way stress affects us. Stress increases our cortisol levels, which affects the inflammation in our body, our sleep cycles, and our energy levels. One way to help lower the effects stress has on our body is to meditate.[6] Do it for any length of time—anything is better than nothing.

Our bodies are warriors that work to defend us 100 percent of the time, but everyone's system is different. We eat different foods, drink different beverages, and take different supplements, antibiotics, gas medicines, prescriptions—the list goes on. It could take a while to get your body balanced so keep going. It does happen. During this time, don't compare yourself to others: this is your journey.

TAKING ACTION

Go with your gut. I can eat oats. Some of you can't. We don't have to eat the same foods; we don't even have to like the same foods to be friends. We can respect each other's choices and wish each other well. Today, pay attention to what you are eating and how your body is responding to those foods.

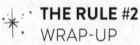

THE RULE #2
WRAP-UP

I want you to eat what you love and allow yourself to get hungry every two to three hours. I don't want you to stay hungry—just get hungry. With practice, you will be figuring out how much food you need.

Eat What You Love

Eat what you love and do not label your food. If you want to change, you must trust this process. Start by giving yourself permission to experiment with foods that you "think" you love. Over time, trust that the choice that's better for *you* will become the more appealing choice. Your body will tell you, but will you listen?

Eliminate Foods That Don't Love You

If you have been suffering from any digestive distress, take a food sensitivity test. Do the foods on your list affect you? If they do, and you know they can hurt you, you now face a choice and an opportunity. Will you keep eating these foods? Maybe at first, but if you continue to experience symptoms, I promise that you'll eventually stop.

Don't Forget Rule #1

Eating what you love only works if you eat when you're physically hungry. Remember that rule also says to start with half of your normal portion and wait fifteen minutes to see how you feel. If you eat more than you need, your body will make up for your mistakes by not getting hungry as quickly. The rules all work together. You can't pick and choose which ones you want to follow.

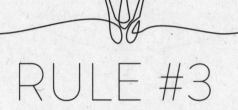

RULE #3

EAT WITHOUT DISTRACTIONS

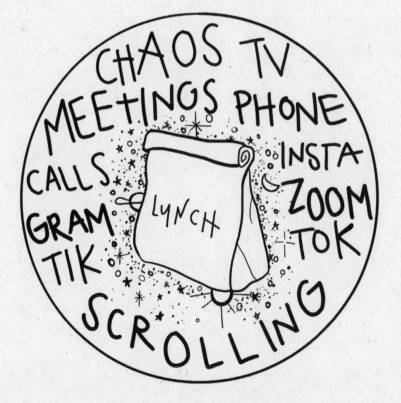

✳ 7 ✳

EAT WITHOUT DISTRACTIONS—
FOOD IS BORING

Rule #1 helps you identify physical hunger. It will help you get in touch with why you are eating and allow food to take up only one important role in your life— fuel for your body. Rule #2 gives you an opportunity to be an authentic eater and to honor your body. This allows you to get unstuck from food labels and judgments about certain foods and find foods that make you feel your best.

That brings us to Rule #3: do not eat while you are distracted. Everyone has one rule that feels harder than the others, and this one I believe is the hardest. You may not agree, but consider the realities of our world: we are so distracted; we spend 47 percent of every waking hour looking for stimulus.[1] The results of the study that found that breakdown also showed that distraction is a mind game. If we focus on how we want to feel instead of how we don't want to feel, we can eliminate distractions. So I am going to give you tools to rewire your mind to shift your attention and focus to the here and now.

You already know from chapter three (part of Rule #1) that it takes fifteen minutes for our bodies to tell our minds we are satisfied after we eat. If you eat while you are distracted, you will miss those internal messages from your stomach to your mind, and you will overeat.

You have also learned that if the food is in front of you and you are not thoughtful, you may mindlessly put food in your mouth—what I call walk-bys, the see-food diet, or fishing. Plus, let's not forget emotions have a way of quickly causing us to impulsively lose track of our plan.

I often hear from people that their biggest problem in losing weight is that they love food too much. So I say, "Prove

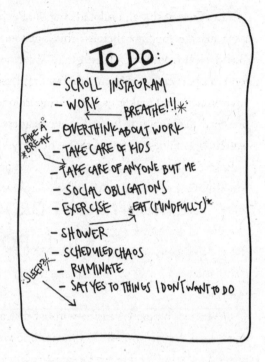

it!" Give your food your undivided attention. By forcing yourself to make your meal the main event, you will eliminate mindless munching and drive-by eating. Instead of grabbing a handful of chips as you walk by the snack cabinet, take a plate of chips to the table and enjoy them properly. When you eat distraction-free, your first revelation will be that food is actually . . . boring. It is the experience of escaping with your partner for a reality TV night on the couch or the atmosphere of a dinner party with old pals that brings us joy. So why do we credit edible inanimate objects with our happiness? The food is just . . . food.

I had a client who wanted to lose forty pounds. She was a binge eater and claimed she just loved food too much. She once reported ordering a frozen yogurt and then scratching her head in wonder, trying to remember who ate it. It was in her hand but she had no memory of eating it. She was too distracted because she was at a baseball game, enjoying the game. If you love food, then enjoy your food. Taste it, experience it, remember it. So if you are going to eat something, focus on it.

Let's revisit this autopilot idea again. People think that their eating behavior is because the food is delicious. This is just not the case. A psychology professor, David Neal from USC, found that "when we've repeatedly eaten a particular food in a particular environment, our brain comes to associate the food with the environment and makes us keep eating as long as those environmental cues are present."[2] Neal's study looked at moviegoers who typically ate popcorn while watching a movie and found that it made no difference if the popcorn was stale or fresh. He gave the participants week-old popcorn. They ate the popcorn anyway. In another study, participants were given bottomless bowls of soup that refilled automatically without them being aware. These participants consumed 73 percent more soup, yet they did not believe they had consumed more, nor did they perceive themselves as being fuller.[3] Both studies are consistent in findings that we will eat more while we are distracted and/or if there is food in front of us.

We need to practice eating without distractions so we can change our habits and wake up our minds. Let me remind you that first you need to be willing to see how you feel when you eat. That's when the real work can begin. This rule will help you cut down on binge eating and overeating and get you to really focus on eating what you love when you are hungry.

Mindfulness is awareness in the present moment. It's being able to observe your thoughts without feelings or judgment. Being mindful is also a way to lower your cortisol level, as I mentioned before. When we remove the distractions (texting, emailing, social media, homework, television, talking on the phone, driving) and focus on why we are eating and what we are eating, we will eat less. And this will inevitably lead to fewer digestive issues, more weight loss, and more satisfaction.

The problem is that there will never be any shortage of distractions, which is the reason why this is also the most difficult rule for people to follow. How many times have you told yourself that you were only going on Instagram for a minute—and then looked up to realize that a half hour had gone by? The exact same thing happens with food. We aren't paying attention, and the food is right in front of us, so we overeat. Or we aren't checking in on what is happening with our emotions and then suddenly find ourselves eating when we're not hungry.

TAKING ACTION

Consider these tips to prevent distracted eating:

1. Find a quiet place to eat.
2. Put away your electronics for a few minutes and resist the urge to multitask.
3. Take a deep breath and make sure your mind is in this moment and that the hunger you feel is in your stomach.
4. After each bite, put your fork down, take a sip of water, wipe your mouth, and think about how the food tastes.

This rule requires the most work, but once you master eating without distractions, you will have made a giant stride in your relationship with food because you will have taken back control and regained any power you might have lost over the years.

YOU ENJOY THE ANTICIPATION MORE THAN THE FOOD

Paul is sixty-nine and a badass in life. He loves food and calls himself a foodie, so when he started preparing his own meals at home, he went all out. For dinner, he made an elaborate salmon dish, really putting in the time. I saw the pictures. It was beautifully plated, like it came from a five-star restaurant, but it was almost painful for him to eat it. Why? He found it impossible to sit at the table and eat without distractions. The very act of being alone with his food made him physically uncomfortable. Think about that. It only takes five to seven minutes to eat half of your normal portion, yet he wasn't able to do it.

This feeling is not uncommon. It comes down to understanding what we really enjoy about food. Let's break down his experience and see if this is something you do as well.

Paul enjoyed the time it took to prepare the meal, because he enjoys cooking. It smelled great. His mouth was literally watering. He even put time into the plate presentation. The table was set for one, and then he sat down. He put the salmon on his fork. He was excited to put the salmon in his mouth. That resonated with all the receptors in his brain and it's what gave him pleasure. He then put the salmon in his mouth, but instead of putting his fork down to chew the salmon so he could taste the salmon and be with the salmon in the moment, he was already piling up his fork for the next bite. In other words, his mind wasn't on the delicious food he prepared; his mind was on the next bite or, worse, somewhere else entirely. You probably do the exact same thing, but why?

It's because your brain has been wired to find reward in the anticipation more than the actual food itself.[4] And if you can't be alone with your food, there is a pretty good chance that you aren't experiencing physical hunger. You're likely looking for a shiny object to distract you, and food serves as that distraction to numb you. Paul's experience might be different than yours, but the pleasure chemicals we get from a shiny object are the same. Studies show that the anticipation plays the key role in the reward and reinforcement processes that maintain binge eating behavior. (In fact, 75 percent of individuals who binge eat often plan their binge eating episodes ahead of time, using it as a reward.)[5]

No matter if these episodes are preplanned when you are experiencing a negative emotion or any discomfort in your body or if they are more impulsive, there is still time to change your mind. If you are in the middle of overeating or binge eating or just can't seem to slow down to wait fifteen minutes for the other half of your portion, you need to disconnect the food from the idea of a reward. And the best way to do that is to spend time alone with your food when you eat. That focus on the food will help you to recognize the difference between a craving, physical hunger, or an emotional hunger—and will dislodge the association between food and easing discomfort. That can allow you to flip your instinct. Then the reward becomes tasting the food, savoring the food, and enjoying the food. So if you can see yourself in Paul's shoes, now would be a good time to go back to your Wellness Wheel and discover what is being neglected.

Your Thinking Mind

What makes distractions so difficult to overcome is that they aren't always external. In fact, some of the most distracting of distractions are your own thoughts and daydreams, which can be an obstacle preventing you from eating mindfully.

We have more than 60,000 thoughts every single day![6] And all of those 60,000 thoughts are automatic. Did you tell your heart to beat? Did you tell your lungs to breathe? I didn't think so. We don't tell our mind to think these thoughts. These thoughts are different from directing your mind to problem solve or finish an assignment or have a conversation. Our minds are hardwired to keep us safe, to create thoughts based on what we see, smell, feel, hear, and experience.

With all that chatter in the mind, it's no wonder why we get distracted so easily. Throw in any emotional triggers that show up in our day and suddenly we can't remember our intentions. It's worse when we're thinking of something that bothers us because we can't help but worry about it. Your mind told you food was a good idea the last time you felt a certain feeling in your body, and you enjoyed the taste of that food, so you will keep remembering that in your time of discomfort and then repeat the action. It's time to wake up and take back control.

Think of all of your thoughts, the good and the bad, as trains. These trains go in and out of the station all day long. Our jobs are to keep our feet firmly planted on the platform in the train station. We can't stop those trains from coming into the station and we do not want to—remember, some of these trains are telling us to breathe. But we don't want these trains to dictate where our minds end up.

Let's say one train carries the thought *I don't want to work out today*. This thought train can derail your entire day if you let it. You do not want to hop on that train or give in to that anxious thought. Just let the train pass. Slowly, and with practice, you will be able to see the train without it rerouting your day or meal.

I understand how easy it is to give in to the thought and get on one of those trains. It can be fun to daydream, which isn't always a negative, but indulging these thoughts, or getting on these trains, can have disastrous consequences. Before we know it, we wind up two hours later still in bed, our workout forgotten.

You know what I'm talking about. You wake up determined to have a fresh start. At breakfast, you're doing great and following the method, checking in with your body to see how you feel. At lunch, it's still all good—then you get a call from someone who needs something from you ASAP and you forget all about being present. Seconds later, you're in the candy bowl before you realize what's happened. You never saw it coming. You get mad at yourself. You might want to give up. Once aboard one of these trains, it's much easier to stay untethered. You just have to learn how to wake up.

The goal is to remain on the platform. In Rule #1, you already learned the best way to avoid getting on these trains: identify your triggers. When you can identify your triggers, you can spot patterns and see how they might lead to certain ways of thinking or certain behaviors. However, you probably also remember that knowing those triggers is only half the battle, because you will never be able to completely avoid being triggered or slipping into the irrational brain. The other half of the battle is practicing remaining unaffected by your thoughts. That's why your new job is to see your thoughts and even laugh at how your mind jumps right into protective mode. Do a mental ping pong—have a conversation with yourself during which you say, *thanks for the reminder of how we used to handle things*, and then let yourself know you are safe.

✳ 8 ✳

EAT WITHOUT DISTRACTIONS—
BE HERE NOW

As I mentioned in the last chapter, this rule is often the most difficult for folks who claim they love food. The reality is we all love food—in a sense, we are all "foodies." But the people who call themselves foodies, I believe, don't love food any more than anyone else does.

I think they love the social experience, the music, the people, the restaurants, the culture, the anticipation of what they get to eat. It's all so exciting. When I ask them to be alone with their food, they get all kinds of squirmy, until they see that the food is less exciting than they thought. And that they can still have the same experiences without the food.

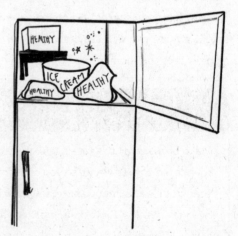

Yes, food may genuinely be a part of what they love about the experience, but it's a smaller part, as they now realize. If you remove all the distractions, the interactions, the music, the social experience, food is really quite boring. That's the very reason why we gravitate toward distractions and entertainment when we eat. Remove that, and we're left with just . . . food. I love food, but I don't need it if I am not hungry. I can eat delicious food when I am hungry and save the rest for later. And this is your goal, too. Not to miss out on pleasurable food and experiences, but also not to overindulge to the point that you feel sad, out of control, or ashamed. Let's remember your rational mind says food is fuel, so if you are thinking food is fun, comfort, entertainment, or the joy in the room, it's because you have been triggered.

Try thinking of the last time you craved a certain food. When you're in that moment, the candy, the ice cream, the chocolate, the chips, the last few bites of whatever it is that you crave feels like the most satisfying thing you can have in the world. The thought of it consumes you; it's like you can already feel it in your mouth, which is why it's so easy to give in. But does that experience stick with you? How long do you remember the enjoyment of eating that food? We have short-term memories. No one can remember the food they craved last week and, without a food journal, the memory of it quickly vanishes.

On average, we eat twenty-one meals every single week. How many of those twenty-one meals do you remember from last week? Probably very few. Do you remember what you ate three weeks ago on a Wednesday? I bet very few, if any, of you will remember. Why? Because it is not as important as you think it is at the moment.

TAKING ACTION

Make of list of all the meals you ate last week. This is a chance to see the abundance of food we ate so you can remind yourself there will be more food later. But it's also important to note how long it took for you to make this list. Even the meals we loved the most are hard to remember. This exercise can help you in the future to remember that you won't even remember that you didn't finish everything on your plate.

I had a running joke with one of my clients who insisted that she could remember everything she ate, so I would test her over and over again. At first, I picked a holiday so it would be easier to remember before asking her about random days of the week. Because it was a game, she fought hard to remember, but she eventually forgot. Do you remember what *you* ate last Thursday?

No matter how much emphasis we put on what we're eating at the moment, we will forget. What we remember is who we were with and what we were feeling at the time and the joy of the moment. If we had a pleasant experience around a meal or with food, we will want to repeat it. There have been many times when I stood looking at the clothes in my closet and thought, I have nothing to wear. Which is laughable—of course I have clothes to wear. And I bought everything in my closet. And I am pretty sure I *had* to have everything. So why can't I remember why I wanted what I am looking at?

That same idea applies to your food—and doesn't mean you can't enjoy your food; your food should be delicious. It means that you shouldn't look to find happiness in food, just like I shouldn't look to find happiness in shopping. You should love what you eat, but it's not where you should find comfort. Food is not the party. It's not fun. It's not a hug. It's not a reward. It's not the tool for numbing yourself. It's just fuel. Shopping isn't my "fun" anymore. I mean, do not get me wrong—I can make a day of it and *have* fun. It's just not where my mind goes when I am feeling emotional. I can't really remember the last time I bought something for the sake of buying it. Just like food is fuel, shopping is necessary. There are times when I need things, but it's not the same as having to have it and having no memory of why I had to have it.

I know that if you've been relying on food to fill this void in your life for a long time, it can feel like you're losing your best friend. That feels sad and scary—but treating food like that is abusive. If you're not hungry but forcing yourself to eat, you're abusing your body. If you choose to find happiness and enjoyment through food, it's probably a sign that you should be having more fulfillment without food. This is the perfect time to go back and revisit your Wellness Wheel. Being well is being in balance. There is no one spoke on the wheel that is more important than another. When you are not moving forward in one area of your life, this lack of progress spreads into all areas of your life.

Look into where that void or neglect is for you in your life so you can try some of the tips I offered in Rule #2 to make sure that food stays where it belongs.

Breaking free from this trap of finding happiness and pleasure from food will change everything. You'll realize that you're having fun with your friends and that you don't need to be distracted by the food. You can be in the moment and enjoy it! If food is fuel and we love the food we eat, do we need food to be our source of pleasure? A better question might be, is food ever as satisfying as we think it's going to be? The answer may surprise you. In the short term, yes, but in the long term, how was that dinner you ate six years ago that you spent so much time worrying about?

ALONE TOGETHER

Think about going to a restaurant by yourself. Would you just sit down, eat your food, and leave? Unlikely. You might feel awkward, so you'd pull out your phone, find something to read, watch the TV on the wall. You'd probably do anything possible just so you *don't* have to be alone with your food. And you've likely been doing something similar every time you eat—finding a way to not be alone with your food, to not feel like Paul from the last chapter.

But the best way to eat without distractions is to learn how to be alone with your food. Before you freak out, know that this isn't forever but just an experiment until you can recognize that it takes only a second for you to assess how much you need to eat, and follow through with that plan. This is your chance to get curious. You say you love food; I am challenging you to see if that's true. Sit at a table, literally alone with your food. Remove all possible distractions. The idea is to get in the habit of setting clear intentions for each meal and not to eat mindlessly just because the food is in front of you or because it's just more fun to eat than not to. I urge you to try it so you can learn to create fun habits that don't feel like chores, so that using your inner power doesn't resemble a self-control decision. Remember, this is about getting curious and creating sustainable change, so keep your focus on the here and now. It's okay to remind yourself that not every moment will be pleasurable and that food isn't always what we need in the moment. Sometimes we just need to breathe and let the moments pass.

TAKING ACTION

Can you pick one meal this week to put eating without distractions into practice? One meal where you eat alone with just the food you love. This experiment only needs to be done once or twice for you to gain an understanding
of why you are eating. Follow these guidelines:

+ Put away your phone, books, or computer.
+ Turn off the television.
+ Cut the music.
+ Get away from the kids.
+ Monitor your emotional state (negative energy, excited energy,
  stress, boredom, and so on).

Even the person sitting across the table from you is a distraction. It doesn't
matter if it is the love of your life, your child, your best friend, or a business
partner, it can still feel like you're being policed, rushed, watched, criticized,
judged, or stressed. The problem with distractions is that they take us away
from our food. In other words, they take our mind out of our bodies, which
means that we're more prone to eat without acknowledging what our bodies
need. And when you eat without this awareness, you're more likely to overeat.

When sitting alone with your food, understand its true purpose and how
it's essential to fuel your body when hungry. You can love how it tastes, but
remember that food is not comfort or joy or even a celebration. Food is fuel.
Take this lesson into each and every meal. Everyone is talking about mindfulness these days. It means being in the moment and having a singular focus.
Mindful eating is the same thing—being totally present and one with our food.

As I have mentioned before, we cannot control the storms in life; we also
can't always predict them. With a solid understanding of your triggers, you
might be better equipped to remain unaffected in the moment the storm strikes.
Today is the perfect day to start working toward being unaffected. I am going
to share with you my favorite things to do to help me stay balanced. Again, it
might sound simple, but get curious here and test yourself.

1. Breathe—take ten deep belly breaths. Picture a balloon in your lower stomach and, with every inhale, blow that balloon up. This ensures you're carrying your oxygen to all of your organs. If we only breathe to our diaphragm, it causes a more anxious feeling.

2. Hum—this sends a vibration down your vagus nerve, relaxing you.

3. Go out in nature—inhale the air, feel the sunshine, and find gratitude for the abundance around you.

4. Meditate—start with thirty seconds, and add more time every day. Get in the routine of doing this at the same time every day.

5. Turn off your phone and spend time with your pets.

6. Just walk—if possible, combine this with number three and walk outside.

These are a few of my favorite things to do. Relaxation, or a calm body, is important for your well-being. And it can happen instantly, just like we can be triggered instantly. With practice you begin to see that the you that exists when you're distracted is linked to many of the behaviors that cause you to give up on yourself and your goals.

I challenge you, especially the foodies out there, to turn off all of the distractions and be alone with your food. Sit and think about your appetite and the ingredients in the meal. Think about where it came from and how it came to be your meal. Are you really hungry, or are you feeling something else? Is the food simply making the moment more pleasurable?

TAKING ACTION

Before you eat, be thoughtful of how you want to feel after you are finished with the meal. Scan your body and figure out what it needs before you dig in, and follow through with this plan. Wait fifteen minutes and rescan to see if you need more. Pay attention to any thoughts you might have and let them pass without engaging. Remain unaffected. This might feel unnatural at first, but find structure in the rule—stick to it and soon it will become automatic.

EAT WITHOUT DISTRACTIONS—STOP AND SMELL THE ROSES (AND THE PASTA)

What's going on around us can change how quickly or slowly we eat, because we often eat based on how we feel. When distracted, stressed, or anxious, we usually eat more and faster. When calm and relaxed, we find it's a lot easier to take our time. Eating without distractions is a rule that's easier for some people than others. When my clients struggle with this one, I ask them to bring food with them into the office, so I can watch them eat. I know. Creepy. But we try to make it as casual and natural as possible. After we get past the awkwardness, I can immediately see ways they can make tweaks and changes to their everyday eating habits. It's usually simple, small things, like not using a giant spoon for peanut butter or not putting a whole pad of butter on a cracker or piece of bread.

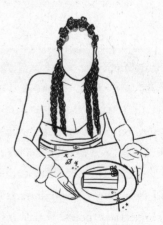

As a reminder, here is a list of very simple things you can start doing today to help you be mindful, so the reward is not in the anticipation but actually in fueling your body.

+ Slow down when you eat.
+ Take a breath between bites.
+ Use your napkin more often.
+ Stop to sip water.
+ Take smaller bites.
+ Put less on your fork, so you put less in your mouth.
+ Eat by yourself (without time pressures). After all, when you're alone with your food, it naturally slows down the process, and you can lose weight from that alone because it allows time for the message that you're full to get from your stomach to your brain, which means that you will eat less food.

Christie is a client who told me that she can't resist the little donut holes they bring to work every so often. She's trying to lose weight, but those donuts are right there in front of her, so she can't stop eating them. It's like a giant rock she's carrying around in her backpack—but there are ways to lighten the load. When asked to describe the experience, she explained how she would pop them in her mouth one at a time, so my first suggestion was to take three bites to eat each donut hole. Slowing down is the first step to discovering what is getting in the way of you actually being with your food.

But slowing down can be scary, and Christie had all the fears in this one—fear of missing out (real FOMO), fear of not having enough, and fear that she will never have them again. Fitness experts remind us often in the middle of pushing us further than we thought we could go that our minds give out before our bodies.[1] If we rely on willpower and self-control, we run the risk of exhaustion and burnout. When we are stressed or exhausted, our mind tells our body to slow down. If we practice being slower, we will make better decisions and develop a stronger connection to what we need. I'm not saying you can't eat three donut holes. I'm asking you to change the way you see a donut hole. To a mouse, that donut hole would be enormous. Try adjusting the lens through which you see food. That doesn't mean eat like a mouse! It means finding grat-itude in what you do get to eat. And why not grab a donut hole for later, just to calm your mind? I bet you forget about it.

As we've discussed, it's not about what you eat, it's about when you eat and how you eat. Learning how to eat mindfully, slowing down the process, and allowing your body to tell you that it's satisfied are all small victories that will add up over time. Basketball players want the ball in the net, but it's really about how they get the ball in the net. How they pivoted and managed to keep focused even though there were many things that could have gotten in their way. If you want bread, then enjoy that piece of bread. Put it in your mouth. Be with the food. Chew your food. The point is to slow down and let the saliva in your mouth do its job.

THE MORE YOU PAY ATTENTION, THE EASIER THE RULE BECOMES

When difficult situations catch us unprepared, we make mistakes without thinking. To avoid this, you need a plan. It's all about retraining ourselves, so we can move forward with new habits. Keep in mind what you learned during the challenge of sitting alone with your food: food is delicious and nourishing; we don't need as much as we think; and it only solves the discomfort of hun-ger. Bring that lesson with you. Here are a few simple guidelines that can help you develop those new habits that will ultimately allow you to see food as fuel, making space in your life to find new ways to find comfort, joy, and happiness:

- ✦ Don't eat standing up—sit at the kitchen table.
- ✦ Don't eat in bed—try reading.
- ✦ Don't eat in front of the television—use a weighted blanket.
- ✦ Don't eat when you walk into the kitchen—grab a cup of water.

Question: Okay, so where can I eat?

Answer: When given the opportunity, sit down. It's that simple. Retrain yourself to only eat at the kitchen or dining room table. If you and your family ate on the couch in front of the television, that's okay, but stop now. (If you're a parent, remember you are also training your kids who will take these lessons into their lives and repeat your behaviors.)

Why? Think about it. Sitting at a table prevents you from grabbing food in the kitchen and unconsciously snacking. It prevents you from mindlessly eating snack foods (or any foods) when you're standing around, watching television, or reading. It forces you to check in with your body, understand what you're feeling, and determine if you are experiencing physical hunger. Get in the habit of checking in with yourself before you eat, while you eat, and after you eat. It takes a second to recognize if you have to pee. The same is true with hunger. This will be difficult at first because you aren't used to it, but you can't keep doing the same thing you were doing before and expect different results.

Don't worry, once you get in the habit of checking in with yourself before you eat, it will become automatic. You can then use that second to make a judgment call. Keep going back to the question, "Am I experiencing physical hunger?" And if you aren't hungry, don't eat, because your body doesn't need it. The underlying problem of overeating is not the food; it's about why you are eating the food.

Hacking the System

Think of the human mind like our control center. It's responsible for every breath, heartbeat, blink, thought, emotion, and our ability to learn.[2] Scientists tell us that our thoughts come from things we see, smell, feel, or hear, or even from a previous thought or memory.[3] It's impossible to keep track of and monitor all the 60,000 thoughts per day that I mentioned in the last chapter. That's why the goal in this section is for you to start training your mind muscle.

Try labeling your thoughts simply as a thought. Here's how you do it. Set a timer on your phone for one minute. Close your eyes and just pay attention to what appears. Some people get bored, or say they don't have any thoughts at all, but if you really pay attention, you will learn that you're always thinking.

I feel great after exercising. – That's just a thought.
I am not having any thoughts. – Thought.
I just want to lose weight. – Thought.

I need to add milk to my grocery list. – Thought.
I have to pee. – Thought.
I need to fire someone. – Thought.

Watch your thoughts like you would a television show. When you examine your thoughts, you can better recognize them for what they are and make what was once invisible, visible. And once you label the thought, it loses its power and disappears. The trains will keep coming. But watch and you'll notice there is another train right behind it. So the next time you have a thought telling you that a cookie is a good idea, instead of getting on that train and wondering how you ended up in a different city eating a cookie, you can label that thought, recognize it for what it is, and move on. When you're distracted and your mind is untrained, it's easy to act on the thought, eat the cookie, and get rerouted from your journey. Our minds are trainable; we can learn and grow at any age. It just requires practice to build and maintain this newfound skill.

This technique allows you to put space between a thought and acting on that thought. This is the point of the entire book—that space between the thought to eat and the action to do it. You will be able to recognize a negative thought or a bad idea for what it is. The thought of eating the cookie is just a thought; it's just your mind responding to what you feel, see, and hear. It's okay to coexist with the idea you love cookies and also not eat cookies right now. Especially when you trust they will be there later when you are hungry.

Labeling your thoughts also allows for space between thoughts, space where you can add your own intentional thoughts—ones more aligned with your *why*. There's a lot of chatter going on in the mind. When you take a moment to stop and pay attention, you'll learn that you have the ability to change the conversation. You might also learn that food isn't what you actually need after all.

THE SEDUCTION IS REAL

A while ago I was having a conversation with a recovering alcoholic. She was telling me a story of how she was at lunch with a group of friends when a random thought popped into her head: *some shots with lunch would be a great idea.*

The thought that shots would be a good idea might not be appealing to many other people at lunch, but to a former addict it was a very seductive temptation. At that single moment, she was at a crossroad. Well, technically every moment is a crossroad, but this one could have 100 percent rerouted her whole life. One way was the habitual, comfortable road to follow, but it was also the path full of worry, sickness, and being unwell. The other way was an open road that led to peace and health and well-being. This path is always available to you; it just depends on when you want to take it.

Instead of acting on that thought of *a few shots are a good idea*, she stopped. Then she whispered under her breath, "Shots with lunch are never a good idea." And then she carried on like it never happened. My understanding was that she was able to put space between her thought and her actions. That space allowed her to laugh at the absurdity of it.

Temptation comes in all different forms. For this person, it was alcohol. For others, it can be drugs; for others, sex. For you, it might be food. For me, it was shopping.

One afternoon while I was in the middle of my own personal storm, I checked my email and saw that my favorite clothing line had a new fall line out—what's more, they were promoting 50 percent off the new line. This was like flashing a new diet in front of a yo-yo dieter, like saying here's a new diet and this one is healthy. Basically, the email created a flood of new trains that were just about to reroute me. This happened to be in the middle of the pandemic when we had all been wearing sweats, so the email pinged all my reward receptors. After all, it had been a good ten months since I had bought anything other than food, Lysol, and tie dye.

That email triggered a reaction in me that had me desperately wanting to click on the link. As I mentioned, I was weathering my own storm at home and not being mindful, so I wasn't even aware I was in a storm. We had sold our house and had thirty days to find a new house and move. I have three kids and a husband, and all five of us were home, Zooming all day long. With three dogs, where in the world were we going to move and how was it going to happen? I had no help at home; we were in the middle of a pandemic. My husband was telling me to calm down, and I was getting more worked up.

So the email was basically a very shiny object that was way more fun than the way I was feeling at the moment. I took this exciting train all the way to the checkout before I realized my alarms were going off. And then I laughed and told myself to hold on—I had been training my whole life for this moment.

So instead of clicking on the link, I stopped to put space between my thought and the action. I checked in with my body. At that moment my chest was tight and restricted. I recognized the temptation for what it was. A minute earlier, shopping had been the last thing on my mind. I didn't need to buy anything. Especially not a sweater that would show up a week later, at which point I would not even understand why I bought it. It most definitely would not have solved my moving problems. I reminded myself there is a sale every week and I could always buy this sweater later if I needed it.

Now with the proper perspective, I deleted the email and honored what I really needed to do at that time. I pulled out my yoga mat and put on some music. Once I started to relax, I became more rational. My husband had been right; I was anxious. I was anxious because I was afraid, but once I was able to see clearly, I found a way to trust it would all work out. And that I had everything inside of me to survive this moment. And it did work out. I never did go back and buy that sweater.

Resisting temptation requires you being uncomfortable at times, but when you put space between your actions and thoughts, and decide not to act on that temptation, you learn that the moment will pass. That is an incredibly empowering moment of truth that builds inner power.

Once you learn how to separate your thoughts (*food is a good idea*) from your action (eating), you can then learn how to develop a way to check in with yourself when this alarm goes off and ask, *Am I okay?*

Rebounding Bag

If you can't prevent yourself from avoiding that state of mind or getting on the train—which would be Plan A—you want to make sure that you get yourself out of that state and off the train as quickly as possible, which we can call rebounding. Rebounding is when an alternative plan comes in, and I keep an actual bag for just such occasions.

This bag is something I'm completely in love with; yours should be, too, since we need all the help we can get. Mine is an adorable bag with a flower pattern on it that makes me smile when I see it. This smile actually changes my physical energy by automatically upping my happiness level. So just looking at it changes my energy and the vibration in my body. It's a way of telling my nervous system to calm down. If that doesn't work, I've filled it with a bunch of tools that can help me reset when I need to find my way back to the train platform. Here's what I keep in my bag:

Aromatherapy: I always recommend that you carry a roll-on tube. As I mentioned earlier, it is one of my favorite tools to help me take deep breaths. When you feel your mind starting to wander from your body, or feel that you might give in to temptation, apply aromatherapy, and take five deep breaths. It will relax you and help to reset your nervous system.

Hand sanitizer: When I'm in a bad mood or someone has said something that I can't stop thinking about, I try to wash it off with hand sanitizer. Sometimes, I go to the sink and literally wash my hands to release the energy from my body.

Lotion: When you apply lotion and say nice things about yourself, it's like giving yourself a hug. Think of it like a stress blanket.

Mini toothbrushes: The smell of mint can be refreshing, and the literal practice of brushing your teeth will freshen your mood. This is a tool just to put space between the thought to eat and the action to eat. I am *not* recommending that you use this technique to avoid eating; you are meant to eat when you are hungry and your body needs food. You just want to make sure you are feeling hunger, and brushing your teeth gives you time to evaluate.

Lip gloss or lip balm: Find something that you love, something that smells delicious or maybe even tingles. Let it distract you.

Headphones: Plug into your phone and listen to high-vibration music, as it is a great way to get out of a negative headspace. Certain music creates calming and relaxing feelings. I personally love loud drums, which gets me out of my own head and gets me moving. I completely forget about what I had been thinking of and get lost in the music. So if you can't keep yourself out of the kitchen, try going for a walk while listening to music with loud drums.

Not every technique will work instantly every time. One day, a particular technique might work quickly, and another day it might not. Keep going. The more resources you have in your bag of tools, the better equipped you will be to resist temptation and weather the storm. There are days when you may need this tool bag often and other days when you do not need it at all. Both are normal. The goal with this bag is to find your footing as quickly as you can. Distract yourself by

+ calling a friend.
+ exercising.
+ listening to positive affirmations.
+ watching a movie.
+ reading a book.
+ going for a drive.
+ listening to a guided meditation.
+ practicing gratitude.

The list is endless, so find what works for you. We may not be able to control what we think, but we can control our reactions to that thought. These are all ways to build your inner power and provide yourself with comfort for what you need in that moment so you won't require it from food. When I noticed that my chest felt tight, going shopping, or even having clothes show up a week later wouldn't help. What I needed to do was honor how I felt in the moment and take care of myself. Chilling out with music or doing yoga to relax is more helpful. When you feel temptation causing you to slip into the irrational mind, or you feel yourself leaving your body, these techniques can be like plopping a watermelon into your lap to ground you. Drag that balloon back down, find your mind, keep going.

When you find that you can be seduced by temptation, go back to look at the Wellness Wheel (see page 40). Are you connected to all the important areas of your life? If you find a disconnect, you will most likely find the void that the temptation is trying to fill. Taking a minute to revisit the Wellness Wheel is like journaling. In this case, the prompt is examining each spoke and recognizing what has been neglected. Do your best to help yourself move forward and get unstuck by connecting to what is important to you.

Forge a New Path

It's never too late to start again. Breaking habits means you have to wake up your mind and practice a new behavior. You have to be committed to this practice.

Let's say that every time you walk into your kitchen, you can't help but open the fridge or scrounge through the cabinets in search of food. Maybe you even eat something without realizing it, simply because you're so used to grabbing food as you walk by. Or maybe you just need a mental break from a task and go fishing in your pantry or coworker's candy bowl. These are habits that need to be broken.

Here's a wake-up idea: try walking into your kitchen a different way. Not everyone's apartment or house has two different entrances to the kitchen, but if yours does, force yourself to walk in a different direction. You can even create a pause in the doorframe each and every time you walk in. Try blocking off the old way to remind yourself to create a new habit. Look for ways to break your own mindless habits, so you can finally shift out of autopilot.

Here is another wake-up idea: place a cup of water on your kitchen counter and drink up as soon as you walk in. We'll get more into the importance of drinking water in Rule #5, but this action will take your mind off food and help you be in the moment. Use the six rules to stay structured and grounded in what you're thinking. Drink a glass of water, take five deep breaths to relax your nervous system, and then make a mindful decision. Do this consistently and you will break your habit of wandering into your kitchen to scrounge for food. Pretty soon, that old habit will become as appealing as robbing a bank.

TAKING ACTION

What habit of yours needs to be rerouted?

What is a wake-up idea you can do to make this happen?

THE RULE #3
WRAP-UP

Why not create a different habit that better serves what your body needs? We all get distracted from time to time. I want you to eat and I want you to eat often; I just want you to be sure you are hungry when you do eat. Rule #3 teaches you to eat without distractions. Make sure your eating mind is front and center. Make sure you aren't focused on a book, watching TV, talking on the phone, or doing work. Make sure your mind is in this time zone and your stomach is hungry. Sit at a table when you eat. Put together a bag of tools to help you resist habitual eating and look for ways to ground yourself when you feel that you have accidentally left the platform and boarded a train to an unknown destination.

Become aware of your eating habits and create new ones. Break old habits that cause you to eat without thinking. If you find yourself aimlessly walking into the kitchen and searching through the fridge for food, change the way you walk into the kitchen to make yourself aware of what you're doing and force yourself to think of the six rules.

Remember, food is boring. Food is just food. It can, and should, be delicious, but let it be boring by not placing so many expectations on it. Be alone with your food and work at redefining your relationship by focusing on food as fuel instead of food as fun or comfort or joy.

Get in touch with and get more used to being your authentic self. Some progress is better than none, and small steps over time create sustainable change. Putting it off makes getting the job done harder.

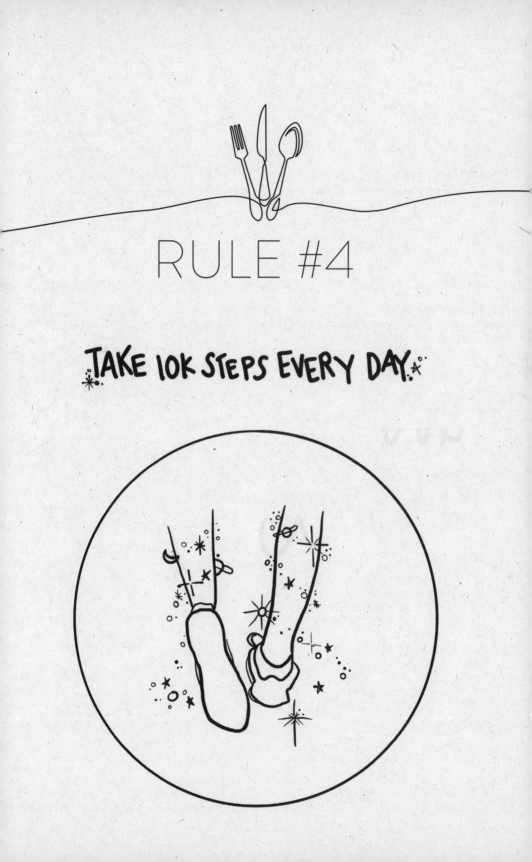

RULE #4

TAKE 10K STEPS EVERY DAY

10

TAKE 10,000 STEPS EVERY DAY— LOSE FAT, NOT MUSCLE

As human beings, we are meant to move—yet so many of us spend all day sitting down. I'm guilty of this as well. When I meet with clients back to back to back, I'm completely sedentary for most of the day, so I know how daunting Rule #4 can seem. Still, if you follow the first three rules, I promise that you will lose weight. And more importantly, it will change your relationship with food. But it will take more than those three rules to help you keep it off.

Without Rule #4—walking 10,000 steps a day—you might end up gaining back even more. I've seen it happen too many times to count. The reason is because losing weight is 90 percent diet and 10 percent exercise. You cannot lose weight with exercise alone. To lose weight, you need to focus

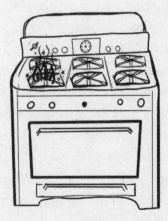

on what and why you are eating rather than how many calories you are burning at a gym (though if your goal is to keep the weight off, the focus changes equally to your diet—what you are eating based on your lifestyle—and your movement. At that point, it's 50 percent diet and 50 percent exercise).[1] But whether you're trying to lose weight or keep it off, the practice of movement should begin immediately. We're not trying to aid in any weight loss—we're preventing muscle loss while also building in a routine that becomes a habit.

The reality is that most people are sedentary, even those of us that go to the gym for an hour a day. Because—geesh!—what is happening the other twenty-three hours? There are one hundred and sixty-eight in a week. I work in front of a computer, so that is about eight hours. I also like to read and watch television and eat my food sitting down. This could be another two to three hours. If we sleep for forty-nine hours and work for forty hours, even if we work out for seven hours, that still leaves about fifty-seven unaccounted hours—most of which we probably spend seated. I think you are starting to see that most of us are really sedentary in our day. A thirty-minute spin class absolutely helps your cardiovascular system and helps you maintain your muscle mass. But it is not enough to call yourself an active person. If we want to maintain our weight loss and achieve a healthier lifestyle we need to move more—and maybe move differently, which is where Rule #4 comes in: get 10,000 steps every day. In fact, the average American walks only 4,000 steps a day,[2] and when you're in that territory, you are more likely to become obese or develop preventable diseases.

Because nobody is going to literally make you count each step you take (how would you even keep track by yourself?), I do recommend that you keep count. I wear a watch to keep track of my steps. If you have an iPhone, the built-in health app has already been keeping track; you can review how you have been doing daily, monthly, or yearly. There are a number of devices on the market that will do the same thing, so you have plenty of options. Find the one that best suits you. I love a device, as it's great for checking your progress throughout the day. Here is a fun fact that can help you achieve your goals: people who track their steps take an average of 2,500 more steps a day than those who don't.[3]

Nowhere does it say that you have to do any of this alone. If you have friends, you can do it together and even link up your devices to challenge and motivate each other. It's an excellent motivational tool. Make sure the people in your life hold you accountable and motivate you to be your best self. I am not saying to ask your friends and family to keep track of you—nobody wants a policeman following them around. But do ask your family and friends to problem solve with you to find ways to promote your exercise routine. You will be so surprised how many folks will want to do what you are doing and will want the same support from you. The important part is taking those steps.

To put it in perspective, 10,000 steps translates to about five miles. I know this sounds hard (don't hop on the fear train!), but it's not nearly as hard as you're thinking. Sure, you can walk five miles in one swoop, but you could also break up the bulk of your steps over the course of the day—and we'll look at how to do that in the next chapter. We will go over in detail how to incorporate getting steps in your day without necessarily upending your schedule, although your schedule might need some upending.

Just as with food, don't look at the steps as being black or white. I think they are nonnegotiable in that you need to take these steps, but there is time to make this happen. They have to happen, but they don't have to happen right this minute; you don't need to start with 10,000 today. Soon you will find ways to move that you didn't notice before. So just look at it in terms of there being room to improve. Not getting 10,000 right out of the gate is not a failure. Start wherever you are and keep improving. Try adding 500 steps a day or 500 steps a week until you reach 10,000. If a client is struggling with the steps and manages to hit a new milestone of 4,000 steps, we can then shoot for consistency at 4,000 before even attempting 4,200 steps. The idea is to keep building and getting more until we can hit the target. We are looking for progress, not perfection, because this isn't going to end; it's going to continue for the rest of your life.

In fact, the Academy of Sports Medicine recommends that we all walk *12,000* steps per day, as this will improve our body composition (body fat to muscle ratio) and reduce the effect on the risk factors of cardiovascular disease (heart attack, stroke, high blood pressure, high cholesterol).[4] But that's a really big goal—the good news is that I have seen the same results with 10,000 steps. While great to shoot for 12,000 steps, our goal is 10,000 steps every day, consistently. And, again, if you can't get there right off the bat, it's fine. Some researchers "have demonstrated that 4,400 steps a day decreases your risk of getting chronic diseases such as obesity, heart disease and stroke. Increasing your steps to 8,000 steps a day resulted in a 51 percent reduction in having a chronic disease."[5] So while we definitely want to make our way to the 10,000-step range, we're getting benefits from moving at all!

There have been multiple studies looking at 7,000 steps per day and higher. Moving is beneficial to balancing your circadian rhythms (sleep and wake times), maintaining heart health, maintaining your muscle, lowering your risk of almost all diseases, and maintaining your weight, to name a few things. If you walk consistently and get 7,000 steps, you are drastically improving your health and reducing your risk of premature death. In fact, "the evidence is strong in suggesting that moving even a little more than before is beneficial to your health. At 10,000 steps you are lowering your risk of death by 40–53 percent."[6] So if you can get more, great, but that's why we're aiming for 10,000. And once you hit that, 10,000 steps every single day is a seven-day-a-week commitment for the rest of your life.

In addition to helping to keep the weight off once you lose it, the 10,000 steps will keep you in balance. Balance means all of our systems are running smoothly, managing alerts productively, and recovering quickly. Taking steps and moving our bodies each day is like offering support to the management of our bodies' chemical activities through something called *homeostasis*. This is a balance of energy in what we eat and drink versus what we use to breathe, sleep, and move. Exercise helps us maintain homeostasis—it helps maintain muscle mass, it helps build more muscle, and it can influence the decisions we make in our day because it improves our mood and our sleep.

Think back to how your metabolism works. Remember the stovetop with the burners? When your body fat is too high and you're sedentary most of the day, those burners won't turn on and you may not be experiencing physical hunger. That's why you shouldn't plop down on the couch and spend the entire day watching television. Those burners start cooling. The more you move, the longer those burners stay heated. Find ways throughout the day to move.

If you start eating more frequent meals (only when you're hungry!), those burners start heating up. Homeostasis is a balance of our energy (including fat reserves), the calories that we put in, and the calories that we use up. We simply need fewer calories to maintain our bodies' homeostasis when we are higher in fat because our burners are not on. Taking 10,000 steps every day will consistently keep the burners lit, which will help you get hungry. To be clear, exercise doesn't make you hungry; it helps in the balancing act. In short, regular physical activity helps you regulate your appetite.[7] Many studies have demonstrated that after exercise we have a decrease in our appetite for one to three hours.[8] And what's more, we have an increase in the mood-boosting hormones that may increase our motivation to not overeat.

There's more: a study in *Health Psychology* found that overweight participants decreased their risk of overeating by more than half when they moved their body for at least an hour a day. The most protective effects against overeating were found in participants who moved or engaged in light physical activity versus moderate-to-vigorous physical activity.[9]

Reminder: hunger is a good sign! Being hungry means that you are activating your burners. Your body is working and giving up what it doesn't need—stored fat. You're not exercising to try to make yourself *not* hungry. You're exercising so that it's easier to *get* hungry.

TAKING ACTION

We repeat history, unless you make a choice to do it differently. The next time you make a plan to meet up with a friend or coworker, be active: skip the coffee date and go for a walk together instead. Can you find new ways to be active?

$*$ **11** $*$

TAKE 10,000 STEPS EVERY DAY—STEPPING UP WITHOUT STEPPING OUT

Stacy is a forty-two-year-old romance novelist. She sits all day long, and she has an arthritic knee, so it's difficult for her to move. Eight weeks ago, she called me, freaking out about her blood sugar and hemoglobin A1C. She's on medication for her blood pressure and cholesterol, and she's borderline diabetic. This cluster of conditions is known as metabolic syndrome, or syndrome X, and it's directly connected to being overweight.[1] Her whole body was breaking down and she was losing muscle tone quickly because she was sedentary and aging, and her liver wasn't functioning properly. My goal was to get her off her meds, so we needed to increase her muscle mass, control her blood sugars, and lower her blood sugar and cholesterol. Lucky for her, it could all be done without restriction.

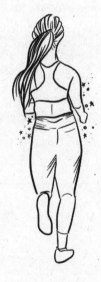

When I asked her what she ate, she said she had no appetite, yet she was still overweight. Notice I asked her what she ate, not if she was hungry. She went on to rationalize her food choices. She told me that her husband was a "healthy" cook, and she snacked on "healthy" fruit (always emphasizing the word "healthy"). She told me she was eating out of boredom and because the food was there, which is common. The key takeaway was that she wasn't hungry. She was what I referred to in Rule #1 as a "walk-by eater." Every time she entered the kitchen, she grabbed a little something.

The first thing we did was apply Rule #1. I asked her to keep some food records for me. I told her to concentrate on the level of hunger more than the food she was eating. Once she started keeping food records, I noticed that she was at the same level of "hunger"—stage 4, ready for a snack—on the hunger scale all day, yet eating different amounts. So we used the first rule to get her to eat appropriately for her hunger level. My goal was for her to understand that even if the food was "healthy" she didn't have room in her gas tank for it. It can't be "healthy" if it's stored as fat and contributing to cholesterol, triglycerides, and blood sugars. So she had to eat less, more in line with what her body needed, to begin to balance her energy, her homeostasis. (This is pretty normal, by the way. If you're overweight, you probably won't be as hungry in the beginning of this journey because you only have a couple of burners on.) As she realized what a 4 on the hunger scale was, she started to understand what her body needed. And as she moved more and ate smaller portions, starting with half and not really going back to get more because she found she didn't need it after fifteen minutes, her body regulated and healed.

TAKING ACTION

Take one or two days this week to track your appetite. Notice if you have hungrier times or less hungry times, or even long periods without hunger. These times will change, so this is just for you to check in and see if you need more or less food at different times of the day. If you repeat this activity a few times, I believe you will see real progress, which is always fun. You will love seeing how your hunger level changes. You will be hungrier as you lose weight and become more active; it's a great sign your body is in balance.

The next thing we did was get her moving, which was the difficult part because it was out of her comfort zone. She had injuries that she worried would get worse, but she started walking anyway. She got to 7,000 steps in record time by deliberately and intentionally walking, and we built on that by adding a little more here and there. After she ate, she would take the time to walk around her condo (whereas before she would sit down to work or read). Then, she started riding a bike. She kept it simple and would do laps around her block. In the beginning she did one lap, and then she got up to seven. (By the way, when I say steps, I do mean steps—please take them!—but I also mean to move your body any way you can. For instance, Stacy could have been sitting in her chair and moving her arms, or lifting weights, while seated; there are lots of ways to move our bodies. More on that in the next chapter.)

After eight weeks, she had lost twenty-four pounds and was averaging 12,000 steps a day. She was eating more often, and even complained it felt like she was getting hungry all the time, and she was loving her activity and the energy she felt from it. Her mood was boosted. She was experiencing physical hunger for the first time in a long time. The burners on her stove had been slow and flameless, so she'd had to eat smaller amounts but more often, and to get moving to turn up the heat. Her body was finally working like it should. Stacy has five more pounds to go before she hits her goal weight, but she's already been taken off two of her three medications.

Excess weight can cause your blood pressure, blood sugar, and triglycerides to go up. Losing that weight can allow those levels to return to normal. By walking and being active, you significantly lower your risk of metabolic syndrome. When we start to build muscle and increase the heat in our burners, our body composition—made up of water, bones, fat, and muscle—changes. Our bodies are made up of between 45 and 75 percent water (sometimes lower when we are dehydrated and sometimes higher when we are well hydrated).[2] If you feel thirsty, you may have already lost 2 to 3 percent of your body's water.[3] This leaves the rest of our weight to come from our bones, fat, muscle, tissues, etc. The fat percentage takes into account both the essential fats (including bones and internal organs) and the stored fat (padding and insulation)—both the fat we need to function and the fat we have in excess that is linked to disease. Fat affects our health when we have an excess of stored fat. Lean body mass consists of your ligaments, tendons, muscles, and internal organs. The reason why we want to have more muscle and less disease-causing fat (though, again, fat itself is not a bad thing—we need fat!) is because muscle holds a lot of stored energy in the form of carbohydrates (glycogen), which is a stored form of sugar (fuel or glucose). When we need energy, our body uses what's stored in our liver or what is stored in our muscles. We only have access to the stored energy in our muscles when we use the muscle or in times of high stress, such as when we have the flu. Higher muscle mass increases our bodies' burn ability, or metabolic rate; lowers our risk of illness; and helps with balance.

Moving your body more helps change your body composition to less fat and more muscle, and releases endorphins, so you just feel better. Your hormonal balance will improve, and your mood will shift because of those endorphins. Endorphins are your body's "feel-good" chemicals that get released when you exercise. Researchers found that exercise "improved executive function, enhanced mood states, and decreased stress levels."[4] That's why, instead of going on a diet plan to lower blood pressure, sugar levels, and cholesterol, we focus on losing weight by following the six rules and becoming more active, letting our brain and the chemicals that manage us become more balanced.

✳ 12 ✳

TAKE 10,000 STEPS EVERY DAY—
ONE STEP AT A TIME

There is a lot of confusion about this topic. The big question always being, "I took a yoga class. Does that count toward my exercise for the day?"

Yoga, Pilates, HIIT, rowing, treadmill, spin, and the laundry list of different fitness classes you can take these days are all great. Yes, you can count them as steps, but these classes alone won't get the job done. I encourage you to take these classes, but do them *in addition to* your 10,000 steps, not instead of your steps. If you take an hour-long fitness class every day of the week, you are moving seven out of 168 hours that week. It's not enough—you will still need to get 10,000 steps a day. I have so many favorite types of workouts that I like to throw into my day if I have time, like WundaBar Pilates (it's so good). I also love my mini strider from Stamina InMotion. If I can't hop on a spin

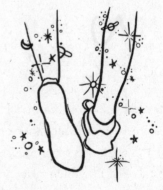

bike or go for a walk, this little machine makes it so easy to get steps indoors, any time of day.

But let's not get ahead of ourselves—you don't need to find your nearest fitness center, take up CrossFit, or go to dance classes while you're upping your step count. We'll get there (when and if you want). But just start with the steps. That's what you want to focus on—and the next couple of sections will give you plenty of ideas for how to creatively get your steps in, and how to add to your overall daily count if you've hit a plateau.

Kayla is a thirty-two-year-old client whose sales job sends her across the country. She's always on the road, and I happened to talk to her when she was in Chicago. She told me that she had the day off before she had to fly to a different city. I suggested, "Why don't you put on your EarPods, and just walk the streets of Chicago? Explore. Go to a part of the city you haven't had a chance to see yet."

That idea sounded luxurious to me, but this was someone who worked so much that she didn't know what to do with herself when she had free time, so she wasn't having any of my advice. She didn't even stick around Chicago. She changed her flight so she could get to the next city early and start working again.

Flash-forward a couple of months when COVID-19 hit and the entire country was on lockdown. Kayla was grounded and work came to a halt. So what did she do? She started walking. Flash-forward another couple of months and she was going on hikes every morning, some for as long as three hours. She didn't even know that she liked to walk before, and then she started doing it all the time.

I can't count how many of my clients have discovered that walking is their new favorite part of the day. Even the clients who fought me tooth and nail about the steps and had been sedentary for most of their lives came around when they made walking a habit. It became their uninterrupted alone time when they can listen to music or a podcast.

You might not like to walk, but I'm willing to bet that there is something out there that you don't even know you'd love because you haven't given it a try yet. One reason a person may overeat is because they are not doing enough things in life they love to do. The more you find that you love to do, the more you can find fulfillment in sources other than food—meaning that Rule #4 will help you follow the first three rules, too.

TAKING ACTION

Take time out for you. Nobody regrets moving their body. Do what you love, try new things, and notice how long it takes for you to love the movement.

📝 Name an activity that sounds interesting to you:

_____

📝 Schedule a time to put it in your calendar and try it:

_____

📝 Can you start adding this activity to your calendar, in short time periods, and make room for it in your life?

_____

📝 Identify the spoke on your Wellness Wheel this new activity fulfills:

_____

Don't overthink it. Nobody is saying that you have to go out there and be a beast. I have those clients, too: they hear they have to do something and then literally think they have to be the best. They are competitive people at the top of their fields, so they go all out and end up hurting themselves or burning out. If this sounds like you, beware. We aren't trying to be black or white. We try to find a peaceful spot in the gray area. The goal is for you to be your most authentic self and to love what you're doing. And if you don't love it anymore, give yourself permission to change it up.

Okay, but, Kim, what if I don't want to exercise? What if I hate exercise? What if I'm not able to exercise? I get it. Exercising has a negative connotation for a lot of people. Maybe you were bullied in gym class. Maybe your knees ache every time you run. Maybe you have asthma. The mental stress associated with exercising is valid.

However, there's no way we're going to let the fear of exercise keep you from shining. We just have to modify the movement to fit your needs. What about dancing to a favorite childhood song? Holding two cans of corn while you're watching your favorite TV show? It doesn't need to be hard or complicated. It just needs to happen.

TAKING ACTION

Make a list of your favorite pastimes—you know, what you used to play as a child. See about scheduling them in. Some examples might be Ping-Pong, swimming, handball, jump rope, hula hooping, basketball—just play. These are active activities that move your body and will put a smile on your face.

Ruth was a client of mine who would fight me on the steps. Some days, she wouldn't even get in 1,000. It was a battle every time I saw her because if she was going to lose weight and maintain her weight loss, she needed to get those steps in. Even on the days she really put in the effort, she might only get 5,000. That was extremely discouraging for her, and it made it difficult for her to keep trying because she often said she went above and beyond what she was used to doing and still didn't even come close to hitting her target. It seemed like an impossible task to her.

To get Ruth back on track, we approached the steps from a different angle. Like most people who had never been active, when Ruth heard that 10,000 steps was the equivalent of five miles, she panicked, because she had never walked that far in her life. It sounded like torture. It's no wonder why people get discouraged and fail. Plus, who wants to do hard things? But the steps are truly easier than you—or Ruth—think, even if you don't love walking. Try thinking outside the box. Here are some simple tweaks you can make to your daily routines to help you naturally get in more steps without even realizing it.

- ✦ Park in the farthest spot in the lot when going to a store. It will force you to take the extra steps to and from your location.
- ✦ Empty the dishwasher one dish at a time. Walking back and forth from the dishwasher to the cabinet will add up.
- ✦ When putting away laundry, do it one article of clothing at a time.
- ✦ Clean your house.
- ✦ Pace while you are watching television.
- ✦ Move your arms during the commercials.
- ✦ Use a restroom on a different floor if you work in an office building.
- ✦ Use a different restroom, if possible, from the one closest to you.
- ✦ Take your dog—or your neighbor's dog—on a walk.
- ✦ Take a walk during your lunch break.
- ✦ Stand during your Zoom meetings.
- ✦ Take the stairs instead of the elevator whenever possible.
- ✦ If you're stuck in an office or at home, pace. You don't want to be sitting for more than an hour at a time. That will help with your hormone regulation.
- ✦ Move the remote when you watch television so you have to get up if you want to change the channel.
- ✦ Go to the zoo with your kids.
- ✦ Pretend to be Dora, from *Dora the Explorer*, with your little ones—run around and hide behind trees like Swiper is right behind you.
- ✦ Make TikToks with your kids.
- ✦ Use a bouncy ball as a chair.
- ✦ Go on family hikes.

I often get in all 10,000 of my steps without having to leave my house. I sometimes spend all day cleaning. After scrubbing my shower and cleaning every inch of my house, I moved 10,000 steps without even thinking about it. These are all small things, and eventually all of those small things add up to big things. Get creative.

Of course, there are nights when I realize that I haven't gotten in all 10,000 steps. That's why I have a little stepper in my bedroom. I can get on that late at night and just read or watch TV while I finish whatever steps I have remaining that day. It's a lifesaver! And there are even a few times I don't hit my steps. I think that's okay, too. I definitely feel better when I do complete them all, so if I miss them, I intentionally shift things the next day to make it a priority. But on those days I don't make it, I don't beat myself up. I am not perfect, but I am practicing my progress.

Find what works best for you. We're all different, with different lifestyles and sources of motivation. When I was sick as a kid, I would have to take the elevator, so I made a promise to myself that when I got better, I would take the staircase. I still do that to this day (and my kids aren't super happy about it). I just refuse to go in the elevator. If my body can do it, I will take the stairs. When I was pregnant and going to the hospital for a checkup, I took the stairs. I get in many extra steps simply because I'm hardwired to take the stairs. You'll be amazed by how quickly you can create that habit.

TAKING ACTION

To change, we need to take different approaches. Try this: at night, most of us chill out, read, or watch television. Why not finish your steps? Better yet, find a way to get your steps while doing what you would normally do. Write down at least three things you can try this week. Here's an example:

1. Pace your bathroom while brushing your teeth.
2. Use your hands more often when you are talking.
3. Turn on some music and dance for one song.

Come up with three of your own ideas!

1. _____
2. _____
3. _____

STEPS AS FITNESS

Once you can comfortably get in the habit of walking 10,000 steps every day, you can look for ways to exercise in addition to those steps. It doesn't matter what you weigh or how many pounds you've already lost, 10,000 steps are the minimum you need to get. If you can't yet, you need to work up to it.

Taking 10,000 steps is what is going to keep you healthy, but if you're looking to get a six pack or sculpted arms or defined calves, you should look into various other forms of activity. I like a little of everything. Don't let this overwhelm you; you will get there when you get there—and only if you want to. Remember there is a difference between trying and allowing—and I am giving you permission to allow yourself to first get in flow with the steps and *then* see where you are. What we do know right now is that the Academy of Sports Medicine recommends that you should always be changing the frequency, duration, and intensity of your exercise, so your muscles remain stimulated (and the burners on your stove remain on). There are five components of fitness:[1]

1. **Cardiovascular endurance:** Your cardiovascular system consists of your lungs, blood vessels, veins, and heart; endurance here refers to your body's ability to efficiently and effectively take in oxygen and deliver it to your body's tissues through the heart, lungs, arteries, blood vessels, and veins.[2] Some examples of cardiovascular exercise include walking, swimming, jogging, running, boxing, circuit training, and cycling. These exercises will maintain or improve the way your body takes in oxygen and delivers it to each of your cells.

2. **Muscular strength (power):** Muscular strength helps you carry and lift heavy things. Without this strength, we would be weak. It can change from one specific muscle group to another. A person might have great strength in their glutes (tush) but not in their deltoids (shoulders). This is why a balanced strength training program that targets all of your muscle groups is beneficial. One example of exercise to increase muscular strength is to work with heavy weights. Generally speaking, the heavier the weight, the fewer the repetitions you should take, but

definitely make an appointment with a local trainer to make sure your form is on point and the weight training is right for you.

3. **Muscular endurance:** This is the ability of your muscles to perform a contraction against a resistance for an extended period of time. Rather than just lifting or carrying something for a few seconds, the muscles are used for minutes. A few examples of this kind of endurance are pedaling a bike up a steep incline over a long period of time to develop fatigue-resistance, or staying in a steady plank position for a long period. The focus you put on muscular endurance should be directly related to your health and fitness goals. For instance, if you want to be strong enough to carry the groceries from your car to your kitchen, you should use low weights and high repetitions. But becoming an endurance athlete will require a continuous muscle contraction, which means you should focus on high-repetition strength training. The Academy of Sports Medicine's guidelines state that adults should perform strength training exercises two to three times a week using a variety of exercises and equipment to target all of the major muscle groups.[3]

4. **Flexibility:** This is the range of motion that you have around a given joint without pain.[4] Flexibility is essential at every age but is sadly often overlooked. In my opinion, it is one of the most important. (Okay, who am I kidding—they are all important.) Without proper flexibility, our muscles and joints grow stiff, and our range of motion is limited, which in turn leads to pain and stiffness that will make it more challenging to do daily activities. That can then impact our balance, our activity level, and even our sleep. Fitting stretching-type activities into your day will allow your muscles to work more effectively and decrease your risk of injuries.

5. **Body fat composition:** This references the amount of fat versus water versus muscle mass in our bodies. High levels of fat are associated with adverse health outcomes, such as heart disease and type 2 diabetes. The goal is to maintain your healthiest body composition.[5] Your composition numbers are important in determining your weight and health goals. Working out and getting your steps in will have a direct effect on your body composition, which is great news.

Find ways to love your physical activity, make it *your* time, and only do what makes you happy. Otherwise, you will be relying on willpower to get through the workout, and you will eventually quit. Start wherever you are and just move. If this feels impossible, trust me—and trust yourself—it's not. The reason why you're doing it far outweighs the why not.

THE RULE #4
WRAP-UP

We need 10,000 steps a day—they aren't negotiable—but we don't have to compete or do it the same way. We also don't need to get there tomorrow. You can be a work in progress as long as you just start moving. Start where you are and keep improving. You can do this. Try adding 500 steps a day or 500 steps a week until you reach 10,000. Anything is better than nothing.

These steps will help your mood (a little happiness never hurt anyone) and your cardiovascular health (your heart will thank you); they will help balance your circadian rhythms, which means you will feel more rested, making it easier to go to sleep and stay asleep; your digestion will improve; and all those steps will help you maintain your weight. Not too shabby!

Get creative, find any activity that you enjoy, and keep moving.

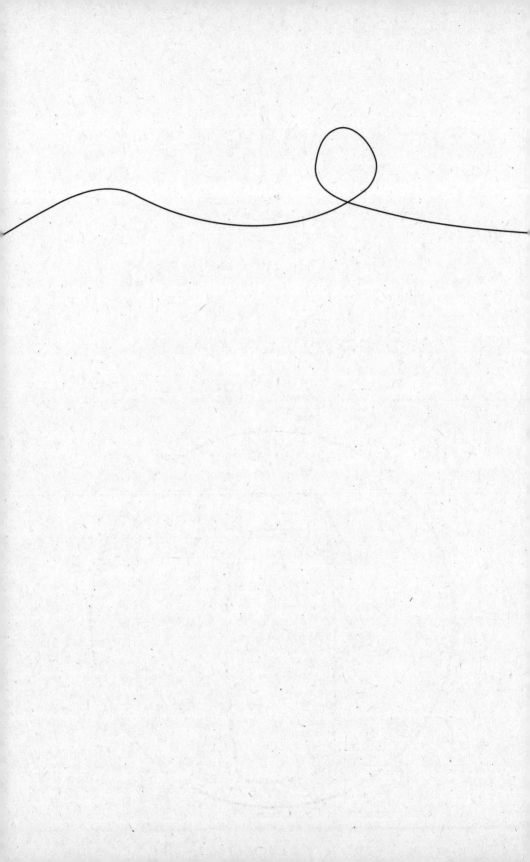

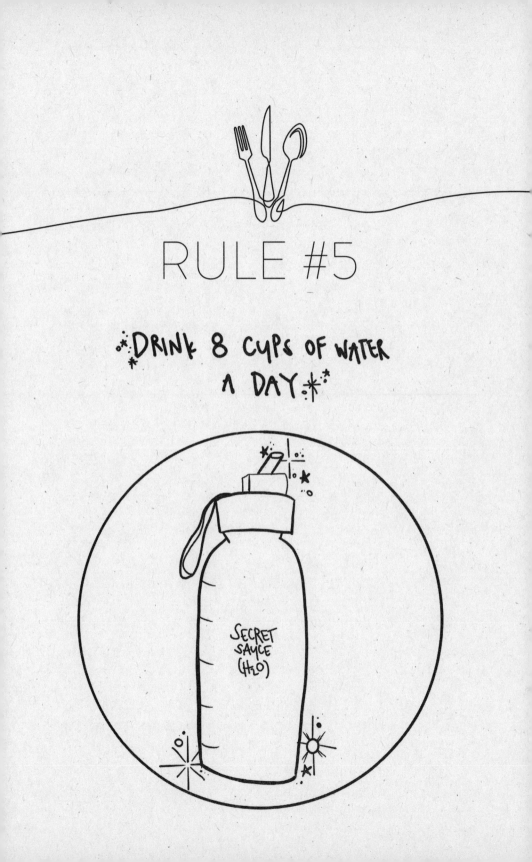

✴ 13 ✴

DRINK EIGHT CUPS OF WATER A DAY—
WATER IS THE SECRET SAUCE

Water is everything!

We are surrounded by water. More than half our planet is covered by water. Water affects our mood and our overall health. Our bodies are primarily made up of water. And this same water is essential for allowing our nervous system to move fluids and nutrients to every cell, regulate our temperature, detoxify us, and hydrate us. And if you've ever wondered why muscle weighs more than fat, it's because muscle contains more water. Our bodies need water, but few people understand how good water really is and how good it makes us feel. We literally cannot live without water. So let's break it down.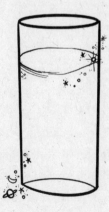

The majority of the water in our body is inside our cells. Our bodies will hold on to water when we don't have enough and will get rid of it when we have too much. A good way to check in with your level of water is to check your pee: if it's light, you are hydrated; if it's dark, you need more water. The body's water regulation is precise. Both water intake and water losses are controlled to reach water balance (and young infants and elderly people are at greater risk for imbalance). Thirst is triggered by the brain's detection that your cells are shrinking—due to lack of water, which we lose through sweat, tears, urine, and feces—and that refreshing feeling after you've taken a long gulp of water is your body's way of filling in the gaps.[1] When you drink water, your body works to absorb it right away.

Nobody can really state how much water each of us needs, just like I can't predict your portion and how much you need at each meal. What I can predict is that you need food and you need water and that every vital organ has different amounts of water stored inside it. We can get water through our food, but this water needs to be digested and absorbed first, whereas the water we drink is absorbed faster. So, for the purposes of this book, we will be focusing on drinking water. There are lots of reasons why a person might need more or less, but per Rule #5, aim for eight eight-ounce cups of drinking water every day. Overdrinking water can mess with our sodium levels.

WATER, AN ESSENTIAL NUTRIENT

Water is used in every cell of the human body. We use water to break down, absorb, and transport nutrients from our food, plus we need it to make saliva, all while controlling our body temperature and lubricating our joints without missing a beat in regulating transportation. Basically, water can move in and out of our cells as needed, carrying or transporting nutrients to our cells, and also removing waste from them. Water helps maintain the shape of our cells and adds cushion to our organs. (Thinking about this makes me want to drink some water right now!)

How is it possible that this zero-calorie nutrient can be so impactful? Part of it is honestly because it has zero calories, which means we aren't drinking unhealthy sodas, sports drinks, coffee drinks, or alcoholic beverages. It's also filling; we eat less food when we drink more water. The mechanisms aren't truly understood, but what we do know is that you will eat less food when you drink water before a meal.[2] Water also increases the rate at which we burn calories. Drinking water helps us become more metabolically active, making it easier for us to maintain weight loss. Drinking about two cups of water before eating was found to increase the metabolic rate by 30 percent. Plus, all of our cells and organs rely on water to move things throughout our bodies. Water moves waste out, lowering inflammation. It removes waste through feces and urine. (Some signs you aren't removing waste well are constipation and bloating, lack of focus, muscle weakness, recurring urinary tract infections, kidney stones, and fat gain.[34]) Dehydration enhances metabolic dysfunction.[5] Another benefit to drinking water is that it's linked to improved skin elasticity—meaning less sagging and fewer wrinkles. Water helps regulate blood pressure by keeping the blood flowing effectively. Hypertension, or high blood pressure, is commonly seen in dehydrated people. When our body lacks water, the brain sends a signal to our body that forces our blood vessels to tighten. If this continues to happen, it causes our heart to pump harder, leading to serious health problems.

Water has a role in our stress level as dehydration can increase the stress hormone, cortisol.[6] High levels of cortisol are linked to obesity. Water can help boost our brainpower—our brains are made up of 73 percent water, so slight levels of dehydration affect our memory and cognitive function.[7]

In other words, water is really important.

What Is Dehydration?

I am sure you have experienced thirst, right? Just like hunger and needing to use the bathroom, thirst comes from signals sent to the brain. When we get the sensation in our mouths or throats that we are thirsty, we know exactly what's wrong and how to fix it. It's also an easy problem to fix. Still, 75 percent of adults are chronically dehydrated and drink only two and a half cups of water a day.[8] Dehydration can lead to:

+ muscle cramps
+ headaches
+ dizziness
+ constipation
+ dry mouth
+ fatigue

✦   weight gain
✦   high cholesterol
✦   high triglycerides
✦   bad breath
✦   joint pain

Dehydration can prevent the bowels from detoxing and cause constipation. High water intake can help prevent kidney stones, lung issues, high blood pressure, low blood sugar, heart attack, stroke, dental disease, urinary tract infections, bladder issues, colon cancer, and gallstones.[9] Often the symptoms of dehydration are a day removed, so drinking more water today will help you feel better tomorrow.

Question: "How can I tell if I'm dehydrated?"

Answer: There are some obvious signs, such as dry tear ducts, or you aren't peeing frequently and your urine is dark when you do. Ideally you want your urine to be as clear as possible. (However, certain vitamins can turn your urine yellow even if you are hydrated.) You can also notice dehydration in the plumpness of the skin in your hands and feet. If your skin is hydrated, it will appear soft and doughy. If you are dehydrated, your skin will lack elasticity and, when pinched, it doesn't bounce back right away. If you don't drink enough water, you can feel tired, achy, and foggy, like you have the flu.

The lungs, digestive tract, kidneys, and liver all eliminate toxins, but if you don't drink enough water, toxins can build up. That means the kidneys can't do their job and you end up taxing your liver, which interferes with its ability to metabolize fat, so the body stores that fat. This can cause:

✦   a rise in cholesterol, which is linked to heart disease.
✦   a rise in triglycerides, which is linked to stroke.
✦   an increase in body fat, which is linked to dehydration and high cortisol levels.

Just by adding water, you help your kidneys function properly and avoid overworking the liver, so you can lose weight and get healthier.[10]

Sometimes we have trouble absorbing water. That too can vary day to day and even hour to hour. The exact amount you need can vary based on your activity, the climate you live in, and what you are eating. As we have mentioned throughout this book, our bodies' internal world is communicating to help us stay balanced, to alert us when it's time to pee, eat, drink, or sleep. And a large part of that communication is done through electrolytes. These little guys are sparks of electricity (minerals, really) that dissolve in water. Everyone needs these little electrical charges to survive. The energy charge is responsible for how water moves around and in and out of cells. The electrolytes in our body include sodium potassium, calcium, bicarbonate, magnesium, chloride, and phosphate. Some signs and symptoms of electrolytes being out of balance, either too high or too low, include:

- ✦ irregular heartbeat
- ✦ headaches
- ✦ weakness
- ✦ twitching and muscle spasms
- ✦ changes in blood pressure
- ✦ excessive tiredness
- ✦ numbness
- ✦ confusion
- ✦ bone disorders
- ✦ nervous system disorder
- ✦ seizures
- ✦ convulsions
- ✦ dry mouth
- ✦ loss of appetite
- ✦ thirst
- ✦ stomach pain
- ✦ constipation
- ✦ nausea
- ✦ vomiting[11]

It's easiest to absorb water on an empty stomach, as then it can quickly pass through our bloodstream, but with food in our system, it could take longer. Tap water and bottled water contain small amounts of electrolytes. Some causes of electrolyte imbalances are not preventable, such as with kidney disease (unless the disease is preventable to begin with), but unless you're losing a lot of electrolytes from heat, sweat, or diarrhea, our bodies do a good job of keeping the electrical currents running smoothly. In my opinion, if you are going to be outside playing a sport for longer than two hours, it's always a good idea to have a small amount of a sports drink during or after to help prevent any imbalances. Like with any nutrient, too little or too much can undo the balance. Overhydration is overdrinking water; although it's not very common, it does happen and can disrupt your water balance, which can impair how your body feels and functions. Ingesting too much water or not drinking enough water will actually feel similar and will be hard to distinguish. Always listen to what your body needs. If you feel like you have an imbalance or have had diarrhea or vomiting for twenty-four hours, consult your doctor.

That said, we aren't a society that generally drinks fluids to quench our thirst. We do it more for pleasure, and unfortunately this has some disadvantages, such as an increase in calories that have a direct effect on our weight. We are not drinking because we are hungry or have room in the tank; it's just for fun. The proportion of water in our diet has diminished over time as we have shifted to a range of beverages that contain either one or many of the following: sugar, caffeine, natural and artificial flavorings, non-nutritive sweeteners, carbonation, or alcohol.[12] (Carbonated water is not usually my first choice when referencing water intake because of the effects it can have on the enamel of our teeth. Carbonated water has been found to have a negative, destructive effect on teeth, leading to a breakdown of sealed tooth enamel resulting in enamel erosion.[13] In addition, carbonated water increases belching and bloating as the body is releasing the carbon dioxide ingested, which can be distressing for some people, affecting their mood, quality of life, and sleep. Still, carbonated water is as hydrating as still water.) All of these beverages are part of our socializing, business meetings, addictions, or sporting events for adults and kids.

Here's the way I see it: a calorie is a calorie is a calorie. We could be talking about pasta and cheesecake or coffee and pastries or wine and Gatorade. No matter what, things with calories only *need* to be consumed when you're hungry. Can you be more selective and choose water more times than not? It's normal to have birthday cake, and it's normal to have a cocktail—it's even normal to have them at times when you're not hungry! It just becomes blurred when we do it every day, when it becomes more of a habit.

Part of having a normal relationship with food is feeling at peace in your body and in the way your body feels. When we drink more water, we perform better in any and all activities. Proper hydration is also linked to our mood, our memory, and our ability to concentrate and multitask. Research shows that just a short period of mild dehydration can suppress blood flow to our brains, impairing short-term memory, reaction time, and attention—and prolonged dehydration can affect planning skills.[14] You can tell if you are mildly dehydrated if you are very thirsty, peeing fewer than four times a day, or if you have dark yellow and strong-smelling urine. Drinking a couple of glasses of water will immediately help this. Some other signs to be on the watch for are dry mouth and being light-headed. Severe dehydration is, well, more severe; it can mean a fever, fatigue, bad mood, headache, and a change in your weight.[15]

What's more, studies have found that drinking about six ounces of water helped with anger, fatigue, and, obviously, hydration status—and about fifteen ounces improved memory and cognitive performance.[16] We also know that drinking water is associated with a decreased risk of depression and anxiety in adults.[17] All of these findings show how important water is in your journey to being well. By drinking more water, we will make better decisions, slow the way we react to situations, let our organs do their jobs without added pressure, and look and feel better overall. Water might be our secret weapon.

TAKING ACTION

What prevents you from drinking water?

_____

Make a plan to change what is getting in your way:

_____

14

DRINK EIGHT CUPS OF WATER A DAY— EVERYTHING WEIGHS SOMETHING

Yes, the goal may be to lose weight, but contrary to popular belief, the scale is not your enemy. It's a great way to read where you are right now. However, don't get caught up on the number because there are so many factors that go into your weight that it might not be an accurate depiction of your true weight. Daily fluctuations are normal. All food and all drinks have a weight. Urine and stool have a weight. Our hormones fluctuate, and even medications can affect your weight. If you worked out yesterday for the first time in a month, it can affect your weight. A cocktail with alcohol may slow your digestion, which leads to water retention, which can affect your weight.[1] A high-sodium meal you ate last night with barbecue sauce or soy sauce or marinara sauce can affect the number on the scale. That's why, if you

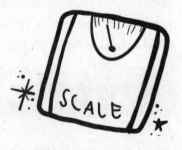

are going to use a scale as a metric, you should be aware there is more going on than meets the eye.

Did you know drinking two eight-ounce cups of water is equivalent to a full pound? Did you just gain a pound? No, you just put a pound in your body, so the scale will reflect that if you were to step on it after drinking a lot of water. Some people like to weigh themselves after they work out, and then call me all excited saying how they lost two or three pounds. No! You just lost all of that weight in water. You're dehydrated and probably feel awful. Go drink some water! You want to drink water during your workout so that you maintain hydration. Ideally, you want to be the same weight before your workout as you are after your workout. If you aren't, you want to replenish what you've lost, or you will be dehydrated.

Let's rethink our relationship with the scale. Maybe you've seen it as a symbol of all your past "failures," or the word "scale" itself is triggering to you. If you decide to use it moving forward, I want you to see it simply as a tool. To be clear, you do not need to use a scale; the choice is yours, and either way, it's okay. For some people, their entire day is dependent on that number they see on the scale, and if they don't see what they like, they feel unworthy. For those people, I recommend that you wean yourself off the scale. We have lots of other ways to determine how we are doing, and it would be so much better if they were positive rather than negative.

But not everyone views the scale as negative; some people like the data and use it to measure how they are doing. For some people, the scale keeps them grounded. But if you're going to weigh yourself, do it once a week, not every day. Pick one day of the week and weigh yourself first thing in the morning after you've peed. That's when your weight is the most accurate. Still, there's a pattern to our weights. Some researchers found that people are heavier early in the week (Sunday and Monday) and their weight decreases during the week. The increases began on Saturday and the decreases began on Tuesday.[2] My theory is that the weekends are the time people are more likely to drink and go out to restaurants, which means your weight is always higher because of the sodium and alcohol, and it takes three days to normalize.

That's why I say weigh yourself on Thursday. In my experience it's your lowest weight of the week. Many folks eat more consistently Monday through Friday. While it is my goal to get you consistent all seven days of the week, let's start with one step at a time. Part of having a normal relationship with food is understanding that eating more than you need at one meal, or drinking more than you need sometimes, is okay. It's never something for which you should punish yourself. What matters is how you feel in each and every moment. The problem comes when a person overeats or overdrinks at one meal, and then think they permanently screwed up and abandon the rules. This leads to inconsistency, which is what causes our bodies to hold on to fat because it fears a famine. It is always best to enjoy yourself within the six rules, of course, but even if you break one or all of them, it's still fine to enjoy yourself and then just get right back on track. Let your body take care of you, trust it to make up for any "mistakes," and carry on.

SO WHAT IS NORMAL WEIGHT?

It's a question I'm frequently asked and one that can easily confuse you with all the mixed messages out there. So let me set the record straight. Your body's natural weight is based on your bone structure, muscle mass, and basal metabolic rate. It's the way you were designed to be before yo-yo dieting or emotional chaos blurred your path.

Your normal weight is your body's healthiest self—where your weight determines your metabolic regulation for cholesterol, blood pressure, blood sugar, and triglycerides. Your normal weight is where these are all in normal range.

Your normal weight is fewer doctor appointments, freedom from worrying about disease, and freedom from obsessing over food.

Have you ever set a weight goal based on a chart? The ones designed to tell us we are "normal" based on only our height and weight? These are important charts in many ways, for sure, but just keep in mind our true normal weight can be plus or minus 10 percent on the ranges listed on those charts. These charts are a useful tool, but not the whole story. For instance, the chart isn't breaking down your body composition. What if you are an athlete and your weight is mostly muscle? The ratio will be off, and you will rank as obese. Plus, the chart can be misleading depending on your age, gender, race, and ethnicity.

Instead of using a chart, I want you just to focus on your individual self—not comparing yourself to any other person. I am sure some of us weigh the exact same, yet we're all different heights and shapes, with a slew of other factors that contribute to how we look. We are who we are. You don't want your goal to be connected to another person's. Keep the focus on you. How and when do you feel your healthiest self? What is the normal weight for you? As we know, our body communicates through signals; sometimes we miss the first few signals and our body has to communicate louder so we can see it, feel it, and hear it.

Take metabolic syndrome, for instance—the cluster of conditions that can occur together, from which my client Stacy suffered back in chapter eleven. These conditions include high blood pressure, high blood sugar, insulin resistance, high cholesterol, and high triglycerides, and they stem from being overweight.[3] Having one of these conditions does not qualify as having full-blown metabolic syndrome, but together your body is saying, *Hey, we need to make some lifestyle changes or we will have some pretty serious health issues.*

So instead of using a chart to determine your normal weight, I would love for you to focus on when you feel the most energy, sleep well, digest well, have a good appetite, and your blood tests from your doctors indicate your body is functioning at its peak level. If your weight has changed and your clothes are tighter, that's not what you should be focusing on. But if your stress has increased, your sleep has decreased, your digestion has changed, and now you have either high cholesterol, high blood sugar (even occasionally), high blood pressure, or high triglycerides, you have crossed a line into what is no longer your normal or optimal weight.

I had a client who restricted herself and then binged. She monitored everything she ate and weighed herself, because that's how she felt safe. We noticed that whenever she would binge, it wouldn't be reflected in her weight on the scale for about two weeks. I learned this wasn't unique to her and her situation. I've noticed that the weights of almost all of my clients were reflective of the last two weeks. That's why the key to success is consistency. And to keep going even if you feel like you messed up. There are no cheat days—because who are you cheating?

If a person overeats one or two nights in a week, they aren't necessarily gaining fat. The reason is because our bodies take about three days to process our food, and eating more than you need is not a consistent dietary pattern, so your body has to step up and respond differently (and it will; don't worry). I have said it many times and I will keep saying it: your body will thrive in consistency. Your body will always step in and try to efficiently and effectively balance you out, but unfortunately over time and with repeated patterns, your body breaks down. If you overeat a meal, and you know this because you feel stuffed at a 9 or 10 on the hunger scale, and you don't get hungry at a 2 or 3 or 4 for many, many hours, it's because your body is working hard to handle the load. Your body will be overloaded with a rush of fat, sugar, calories, carbs, proteins, vitamins, minerals, and water. This will cause minor chaos while your hormone and energy levels fluctuate. There will be information misfires in fat storage, inflammatory responses, and digestive confusion.

Your water balance will be working hard to get back to normal. Sodium will be stored in your cells. In the meantime, you may feel thicker, bloated, and heavier, and it may impact your weight on the scale, but it's not the same as permanent weight gain. Just ignore it. It is in your best interest to not try to do anything other than get yourself back to a consistent pattern. Your body will respond and dump what it doesn't need. If you try to "help" yourself by restricting what you eat, you simply encourage your body to fluctuate more. This inconsistency causes weight gain by alarming your internal body clock, affecting your "hormonal regulation of energy homeostasis and metabolic regulation."[4] In short, never beat yourself up about anything; just trust the rules. We don't gain weight from one meal of pasta; we puff up and then we depuff in a couple of days. Don't let the scale limit your mental success.

You also want to change the way you think about carbohydrates. Carbs are one of the six main nutrients that the body needs every day along with protein, fat, water, vitamins, and minerals. You probably know that carbs are sugar, but I bet you never realized that "carbohydrate" has the word "hydrate" in it. Carbo*hydrate*. Carbohydrates are converted to glucose pretty much the second they enter our mouths. Chewing our food crumbles the carbohydrate and then the saliva in our mouths has enzymes that break it down. Once the carbohydrate is broken down into smaller single chains, it is ready to be transported to the liver. The liver than takes these single chains and converts them to glucose, our fuel. Glucose is than exported to our bloodstream by hormones.[5]

Our blood sugars are tightly controlled. The body has a fuel gauge and internal body clock that keeps tabs on it and fuel in the tank at all times no matter what, without which we could have serious health consequences. In fact, we have about four grams of glucose circulating in our blood twenty-four hours a day, seven days a week. In other words, just a little less than a teaspoon of sugar fuels our cells.[6] If we overeat carbs, then we store the glucose as glycogen in our liver and in our muscle for the future.[7] Each gram of glycogen that is stored is attached to three or four grams of water. That's what hydrates it and that is why you might feel the difference when you cut down on carbs. When we omit foods with carbohydrates, we dehydrate. When you add back an apple, you might feel like an apple: hydrated. And if you are eyeing your scale, the number on the scale might go up, but it's really just water, and that's a good thing.

What happens if we don't work out and don't have a lot of muscle? Our bodies think we need to save it for the future and convert the extra unused glycogen to triglycerides, storing it in our fat cells instead of in our muscles. We want the muscles; we want the storage capability. This is one reason why muscles are important: body fat is linked to different diseases, while muscle mass is not.

Those who eat a high-protein diet don't have carbohydrates or glucose, so they can't absorb water, which means they have to drink much more water. It can be toxic to the brain and kidneys if they don't. When you don't eat carbs (fruits, vegetables, milk, and starches) your body doesn't absorb the water. Our body is up to 60 percent water,[8] so when we go on a low-carb diet it looks like we're losing weight, but we're really only losing water. All we did was dehydrate the body. The second you have something like an apple, you hydrate, and it looks like you gained weight. (You didn't. You just rehydrated.)

I know you are exhausted from the diet industry and trying to figure all this out. But the point is that our bodies are complex and are constantly striving for balance—they will balance themselves if we treat them right. Don't let someone else's weight loss on a low-carb diet derail you. Keep your focus on you and what you feel and what you need.

FOCUS ON BODY FAT

Body fat doesn't lie: every 1 percent of body fat is equivalent to three pounds on the scale. As you are very well aware, a scale can give a false number for multiple reasons, but a person's body fat percentage is *usually* a good indicator of what is going on from one week to another (not always, as it can be misleading based on a person's hydration level). A body fat reading is giving you an estimate of percentages of your body composition. There are different forms of body fat analysis, but I like using a bioelectric impedance machine, which are easy to have at home. This machine measures electric impulses from one hand to another or one foot to another and is based on how hydrated you are. It measures the rates of speed at which one impulse reaches another.

I like using this measure to see *how* a client is losing their weight. When we're losing weight, unless we're diligent about it, we can lose one pound of combined water, fat, and muscle, or a pound of muscle, or a pound of water. But we are looking to keep our hydration status high, and to maintain and build muscle to help keep us metabolically active, so we want to be losing *fat*. That's why it can be so important to know what type of weight loss is happening. Knowing your body fat will put you in the driver's seat. You can help yourself and change your health. You can lose weight without moving your body, but you are most likely losing muscle instead of fat, which is not the goal. Losing weight is great if you want to lose weight, but losing fat is the real win. Losing fat means you are improving your health.

In a single week, it's not uncommon for someone to lose a couple of pounds and not have their body fat percentage change. No need to panic. Remember we have lots of fluctuations, including how hydrated we are from one day to the next. But if your body fat percentage isn't changing, it can also mean you aren't moving enough. So this is your opportunity to step it up a notch with your steps, in addition to adequately hydrating.

Sally is a client who lost twenty pounds, getting her weight down to where she wanted it on the scale, but her body fat remained high at 30 percent. Sally also wasn't a fan of water: she felt like making it to the bathroom was always an issue, and she didn't like the taste. She was already a petite lady, so she couldn't afford to lose any more weight. We needed to change her body composition and manipulate her weight by turning that fat into muscle. The problem was she did not want to change her ways. She had been taking a yoga class twice a week, but that was hardly enough, and eventually I knew that she would put the weight back on. She didn't make the time to move her body. Her goal had been to get to a specific number on the scale; she had never thought about why she was always needing to lose weight, or why she was always gaining it back. In her mind, she reached her goal. In my mind, she had just begun to manage the goal. It wasn't until the pandemic that she started walking and finally managing all six rules. She got in her 10,000 steps, and she started carrying a thirty-two-ounce water bottle. She also loved tracking her progress (I hope you're seeing a theme here). She even started adding other types of workouts such as weights into her schedule. Once she started moving consistently, she was able to change her body composition. She also started noticing that if she started with water at the times she thought she was hungry, it took away her desire to eat. Sally had not been hungry, and adding water helped her know and feel the difference. And this has helped her improve her mood, sleep, and health.

The scale isn't always the answer. It is one tangible marker, but there is more to the story. So if you use a typical scale, maybe ditch it and get one that tells you your body fat percentage, since this is the number to focus on.

✳ 15 ✳

DRINK EIGHT CUPS OF WATER A DAY—
EIGHT CUPS? HOW?!

For some people, drinking water is easy. For others, it's a struggle. Athletes and those who regularly work out usually don't have a problem with this rule, but it can trip up some people because so few of us do it naturally. Digestion issues such as feeling bloated or suffering from nausea or heartburn can make it difficult to get the water down; and drinking water when having loose stool can seem to make it worse. Many clients resist drinking water because they want to avoid frequent bathroom trips, or they worry about making it there in time. Others are so used to getting all their fluids from iced tea, coffee, and diet soda that they find the switch to water undesirable. I've heard every reason and excuse imaginable.

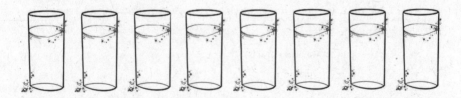

But those excuses are just that—excuses. We can potentially go weeks without food, but we can't survive more than three days without water. If the other benefits were not enough to motivate you, consider these:

+ You are lowering your sensitivity to pain.[1]
+ You can thin mucus if you have postnasal drip.[2]
+ You will have an easier time with digestion and less heartburn.[3]
+ Your teeth and gums will be healthier because water keeps your mouth clean.[4]

If drinking water is difficult for you, you must find a way to make it a habit. Water is one of the most talked about nutrients. I often hear, "I can't drink water, it's boring, I don't like the way it tastes, I'm not thirsty," to name a few. If this is how you feel, I get it. It still doesn't change the fact it's important. How can you make drinking water fun and a challenge that doesn't feel like a restriction? First, you can start with where you are and add a little more every day. And if you can get curious and find fun ways to make it happen, you will see the benefits soon enough—and that will make it less tempting to skip the water. Drinking enough water is a game changer for your health. Here are some more tricks to get started:

+ Drink a glass of water immediately after waking up.
+ Set timers on your phone periodically throughout the day as a reminder.
+ Keep water on your desk.
+ Make sure the water temperature is to your liking.
+ Try drinking one to two cups of water before you eat.
+ Drink a full glass of water before you start doing any mental work.
+ Take breaks to drink water.
+ Add mint, lemon, or cucumber to a pitcher of water and have it handy during the day.
+ Get an accountability partner.
+ Start a water challenge.
+ Set reminders.

Make it as easy for yourself as possible. Take an honest assessment, so you can better understand what's holding you back, and put a plan in place to overcome those obstacles when they arise. Your body will thank you in ways that you might not even realize.

TAKING ACTION

Honestly answer these questions:

📝 Do you like to drink water?

_____

📝 How do you like to drink water?

_____

📝 How much water have you had today?

_____

📝 What about yesterday?

_____

📝 How can you help yourself to add more water tomorrow?

_____

You can space out the water however you see fit. I like to drink half of the water I need before lunch, and the other half after. However, there are some factors to consider. For example, sleep is extremely important, so you don't want to be constantly getting up in the middle of the night to pee. To prevent this from happening, I highly recommend drinking most of your water before 6 PM. This is a suggestion that should help you with our final rule, Rule #6, too.

THE RULE #5
WRAP-UP

If water isn't your go-to drink, let's work on changing that. Sure, water can seem tasteless and not very fun, especially when we are on a constant lookout for pleasure, but we need water. It really is that simple. Water is a big deal, and hydrating our body needs to be taken seriously: hydrating is essential for detoxing, temperature control, healthy skin, productivity, and healthy muscles.

We need to drink eight glasses of water a day. Learning to drink more water, just like adding steps every day, may require a little creativity. Here are some ideas:

Add one glass of water to your wake-up routine.

Get yourself a reusable cup that is fun to drink from.

Try setting reminders.

Drink sips after each bite of food you take.

Flavor your water with lemon, apple slices, or mint.

Dehydration can make you feel headachy, constipated, tired, and run-down; it can lead to weight gain; and it's damaging to your organs. Make drinking water easy and make it a habit. You do not need to be perfect, and every day may be different; just be patient and stick with it.

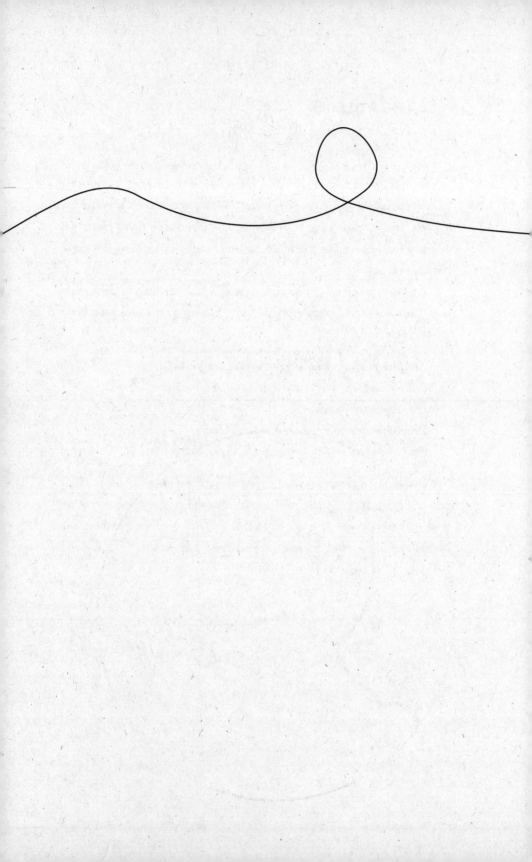

RULE #6

GET 7 HOURS OF SLEEP

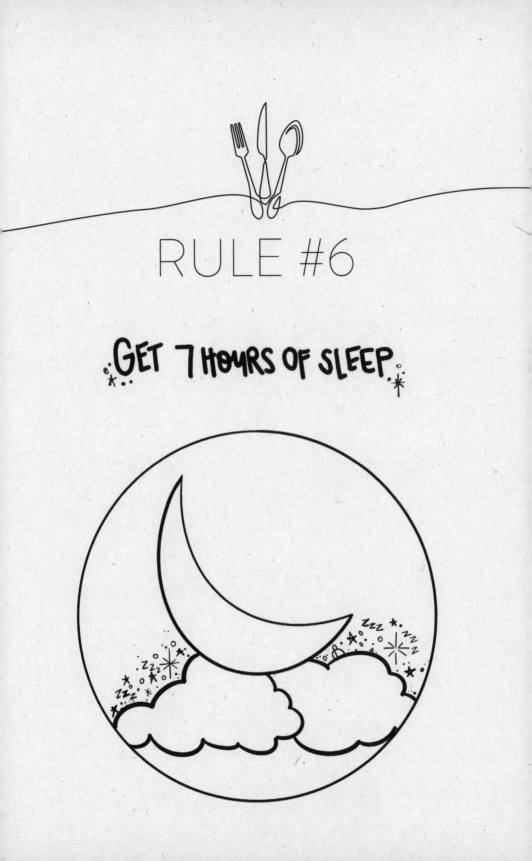

✳ 16 ✳

GET SEVEN HOURS OF SLEEP—COUNT SHEEP, NOT CALORIES

Everyone wants to sleep well at night, yet so many struggle. They try to fix their issues but get so overwhelmed that they give up and accept that they are the type of person who doesn't sleep well. There are up to 70 million people in the United States and about 45 million people in Europe who have chronic sleep problems, and there are more than 100 types of sleep disorder classifications.[1] The problem is that you can't really lose weight, maintain weight, and improve your overall well-being if you are not sleeping well. During the pandemic in early 2020 in particular, it became obvious to me how stressed out everyone was, and how that stress was affecting people's sleep—and how that lack of sleep was affecting people's health journeys. So "Get Seven Hours of Sleep" officially became Rule #6.

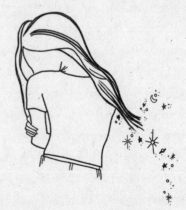

We all need food, water, and sleep to survive and be well. To be our healthiest self, we have to look at our sleep habits. Sleep impacts almost every organ in our bodies. Not getting enough sleep leaves our brain exhausted and our body fighting for balance, which makes it difficult to concentrate and learn and to stay connected to what is really important to us, like eating when we are hungry. Lack of sleep can delay the signals our brains receive and cause us to make more impulsive, irrational decisions (such as *Maybe that chocolate will give me more energy, I need more coffee,* or *I'm going to give up on getting my steps because I am so tired*). Mounting epidemiological data implicates sleep loss as a risk factor for obesity in both children and adults worldwide.[2] Sleep deprivation is considered to be less than seven hours of sleep.[3] Sleep deprivation affects our appetite-regulating hormones and increases our calorie intake. It's just easier to ignore what your body needs when you are tired, especially if you think food will give you some much-needed energy.[4] What will give us more energy is a sleep routine. In short, sleep and the *quality* of the sleep we get is as important in regulating our weight as is the way we eat and how we move our body.

Lack of sleep can also impact our gut. Having a bad night of sleep is linked to higher next-day abdominal pain, anxiety, and fatigue.[5] When we don't get enough sleep, it has detrimental effects of oxidative stress on our liver.[6] Triglycerides and cholesterol increase, which make us more susceptible to infections and type 2 diabetes, and weakens our body's natural defenses, making it more likely we will get sick in general.[7] Sleep deprivation is a little like being intoxicated. Comparison studies between fully rested subjects, sleep-deprived subjects, and legally drunk subjects had some meaningful results: "a person who has been awake for seventeen to nineteen hours is as cognitively impaired as a person who is legally drunk, and sleeping six hours a night for ten days leads to impairment equivalent to a person who has been awake for twenty-four hours, which is worse than being drunk."[8] That's the same as waking at seven in the morning and staying up until about one in the morning. Many of us do that often. It's been proven to make you feel hungry more often, which causes you to make poor food choices and eat bigger portions.[9]

If you find yourself asking questions like, "Why can't I focus?" "Why am I always hungry?" "Why do I only want sweets?" or "Why can't I build muscle?"

and you aren't able to fall asleep, stay asleep, or wake up feeling rested in the morning, there is a good chance that your sleeping habits might be waging an internal war in your body.

According to the Annals of Internal Medicine, getting less than seven hours of sleep per night can reduce the benefits of dieting. Their study revealed that when dieters were deprived of sleep, they lost half as much weight as those who were well rested. Those same dieters also felt hungrier and lacked energy.[10] Even though we're not dieting with the six rules, the findings apply: when we miss out on sleep, we will be more tempted and less connected to our emotional and physical needs, and our bodies will be in survival mode. And in this mode our bodies will protectively hold on to weight because we are telling it that we are in a fight for our life. Our adrenaline will be high and our hormones and electrolytes will be misfiring all over the place. You can't lose or maintain weight if you aren't sleeping.

SLEEP, THE NEW ANTI-AGING SERUM

There is an overall lack of awareness about the importance and function of sleep, so let's start with the science, so you can better understand what's going on inside your body.

Your body's main stress response system occurs through the hypothalamic-pituitary-adrenal axis (HPA) and is regulated by nerves. These nerves are sensors for any and all stress in your life. Your response to acute stress is pretty immediate, and you get a quick hit of epinephrine and norepinephrine, which causes increased heart rate and sweating. This activates the HPA and causes the body to produce a bunch of steroid hormones, which act on multiple organ systems to redirect energy resources to meet real or anticipated demand. So instead of using these hormones to maintain homeostasis, you're using them to deal with stress.[11] Many different hormones come into play in this process, but for the sake of simplicity, we're going to focus on two: cortisol and melatonin.

Cortisol is the end product of the HPA axis. Produced by the two tiny adrenal glands that live on top of your kidneys, this hormone is essential to almost every organ and tissue in your body.[12] Cortisol levels naturally rise and fall throughout the day. Your body is monitoring this hormone all day long to keep it stable because if it's too low or too high, it can be harmful to your health. Levels are highest in the morning, peaking around 9 AM, and drop to their lowest level around midnight before the cycle begins again. This cycle can be altered or affected by many different things such as caffeine, chronic stress, poor nighttime behaviors, certain medications, an adrenal gland tumor, malnutrition, diabetes, polycystic ovarian syndrome, a pituitary gland issue, poor sleeping habits, and alcoholism. Since cortisol spikes during times of stress to help your body deal with sudden changes, it's often referred to as "the stress hormone." Cortisol plays a significant role in a number of your body's functions, including:

+ metabolism
+ stimulating liver function to increase blood sugar production[13]
+ converting fats, carbohydrates, and proteins into usable energy
+ influencing your body's fight or flight response
+ providing an energy boost when you're stressed or threatened[14]
+ fighting inflammation
+ helping to balance the salt and water in your body
+ regulating blood sugar
+ activating the body to make more ghrelin, which is one of the hormones that controls hunger[15]

When your cortisol is high, all of those functions can be at risk. Some signs and symptoms that your cortisol levels are high include:

+ susceptibility to infection
+ autoimmune disorders
+ type 2 diabetes mellitus
+ cardiovascular disease (heart attack and stroke)[16]
+ weight gain
+ fatigue
+ acne
+ thinning hair
+ bruising
+ healing more slowly from wounds
+ weak bones

+ muscle weakness
+ low sex drive
+ high blood sugar
+ irregular periods
+ anxiety and depression
+ arthritis
+ sleep problems
+ difficulty concentrating[17]

And one thing that lowers those levels back to normal is sleep.

Melatonin regulates the HPA so that you can get sleep and have normal cortisol levels; it also plays a role in reproduction and immunity. This is the calm, sleepy hormone that your body produces in response to dimming light that helps to promote sleep. If you are exposed to light in the evening, it can block your body's melatonin production. Melatonin is mostly made by the pineal gland, located in the middle of your brain, and it responds directly to the sun. So when the sun goes down, our melatonin levels go up, thus inducing sleep. We can support our bodies' production of melatonin by sticking to a normal sleep schedule because our bodies thrive in consistency. Melatonin has many benefits that are profound and far reaching, including reducing inflammation and preventing tissue damage.[18] It also delays and perhaps treats age-related diseases.[19] Melatonin may also increase our metabolism and help folks lose weight by improving the health of our mitochondria and by helping turn fat into energy. We need our levels of melatonin balanced—and to do that, we have to focus on our sleep habits. Reasons why we might see a decrease in our bodies' natural secretion of melatonin include:

+ age (our bodies simply produce less melatonin as we age)
+ type 2 diabetes
+ some mood disorders
+ some cancers
+ dementia[20]

One thing to keep in mind about melatonin, though: supplements aren't regulated. A study of thirty-one different melatonin supplements found that the actual amount of melatonin ranged from 83 percent to 478 percent of what was advertised on the label.[21] When it's possible, check your labels and look for National Sanitation Foundation (NSF) or United States Pharmacopeia (USP) as this means the supplement has been verified by experts. But still, evidence supporting melatonin use for sleep disturbances is weak.[22] Melatonin supplementation tricks your brain into thinking it's sunset and turns up sleepiness; it should take effect within thirty to sixty minutes and can stay in your system for four to ten hours, depending on the dosage.[23] My goal is for you to get your body into its natural balanced state so you don't require sleep aids (we will further discuss how to make this happen in chapter eighteen).

Cortisol and melatonin are supposed to have a symbiotic relationship because cortisol suppresses melatonin during the day so we can stay awake, and melatonin suppresses cortisol levels in the evening and at night so we can sleep. It's when that relationship gets thrown out of whack that we can experience sleep issues, so it's all about building healthy habits to get back on track.

TAKING ACTION

Let's see how you are doing. Answer yes or no below.
Focus on how you sleep:

Can you fall asleep easily?

_____

Can you stay asleep?

_____

Do you feel rested in the morning?

_____

If you answered no to any of these questions, we need to work on getting these hormones back in balance.

HOW MUCH SLEEP DO YOU NEED?

Your body clock, or circadian rhythm, runs on a twenty-hour cycle, and influences crucial functions such as hormone release, eating habits, digestion, and body temperature. This rhythm is your body's way of putting you into homeostasis, so, when you fall out of that rhythm, your entire body is impacted. When your HPA axis is under chronic stress, it disrupts your circadian rhythm, resulting in inflammation, blood sugar imbalances, lack of sleep, and mental/emotional stress.[24] A recent study found that women who slept for five hours per night were thirty-two percent more likely to experience major weight gain (defined as an increase of thirty-three pounds or more) over the course of the sixteen-year study than those who slept seven hours.[25] And in another study, men who got "five hours of sleep a night, four nights a week, followed by one ten-hour night of 'recovery sleep' stored more fat" than other men.[26]

One myth that I want to dispel is that we can make up for lack of sleep. If you've been traveling or pulling all-nighters for a couple of days, don't assume that you'll just sleep in over the weekend and make it all up. It doesn't work like that. Sleep is essential. More than one third of American adults are not getting enough sleep on a regular basis.[27] Short sleep duration is defined as fewer than seven hours of sleep in twenty-four hours.[28] I know sleeping in sounds fun and better than feeling tired, but you will still feel tired and your body will still be under fire. In fact, one study found that sleeping in on the weekends doesn't reverse the metabolic dysregulation and potential weight gain associated with regular sleep loss.[29] So even though it might be difficult for the first couple of days, you have to keep striving to find that consistency.

We can't really think of sleep like a checking account where we can make deposits and withdrawals. Taking an hour out on Wednesday and on Thursday and then depositing four hours of sleep on Sunday isn't a perfect solution. Your circadian clock is sensitive; any disruption dysregulates your hormone levels. If you tinker with your sleep times, you will see consequences. Your body likes consistency. If you are struggling with getting more sleep, put your focus on routine and structure: go to bed at the same time every night and wake up at the same time every day. Research has shown that it can take us up to four days to recover from one hour of lost sleep, and up to nine days to balance our circadian rhythms.[30]

So what is enough sleep? According to the Centers for Disease Control and Prevention (CDC), it can vary from person to person and is dependent on age. As we age, we need less sleep to function. Here are the general National Sleep Foundation guidelines:

Newborns (0 to 3 months): 14 to 17 hours
Infants (4 to 12 months): 12 to 16 hours
Toddler (1 to 2 years): 11 to 14 hours
Preschool (3 to 5 years): 10 to 13 hours
School age (6 to 12 years): 9 to 12 hours
Teen (13 to 18 years): 8 to 10 hours
Adult (18 to 60-plus years): 7-plus hours[31]

So you've probably noticed that it says seven-*plus* hours—so why is Rule #6 to get seven hours of sleep? Because progress is better than perfection. Small improvements are better than zero, and if I can help someone get seven hours of sleep, they will eventually get more. The current recommendation for "adults is 7 or more hours per night to promote optimal health."[32] So, basically, we're trying for *at least* seven hours of sleep. Fewer than seven hours of sleep is linked to anxiety, unpleasant mood, and tiredness during the day.[33] According to a six-year study on sleep duration and weight gain, "The risk of developing obesity was elevated for short- and long-duration sleepers as compared with average-duration sleepers, with 27% and 21% increases in risk, respectively."[34]

Jason was a forty-year-old client who suffered from an eating disorder, OCD, and anxiety since he was a kid. He relied on multiple sleep aids to fall asleep, only to wake up at 2 AM like clockwork. His stress levels were so high that he woke fully alert and ready to start the day in the middle of the night. He didn't groggily wake up to pee—he woke up and was alert, with his mind racing. Not only was he awake in the middle of the night, but he was starving, so he binged. Because he felt guilty, he restricted his food intake all day in fear of nighttime binging. His mind wasn't clear, so he made poor choices during the day. And what's more, he pushed himself in his workouts, even when exhausted. All the while, he still couldn't sleep, and the cycle repeated itself.

Fixing Jason's sleep patterns could help improve 90 percent of his issues, so that's what we focused on. We started by trying to course-correct his nervous system because his stress hormones were so high that he was burning out. This required tweaking the timing of his meals, adding deep breathing practices, changing his workout routine to match the way his body was feeling, and adjusting his bedtime.

Jason started with a schedule to eat every three hours to help his body relax. My goal was to balance his glucose regulation. Since eating signals the body it's time to get to work (digest and absorb), and we want our body to do this kind of work during the day, if we eat close to bedtime or wake up and eat, it wakes up our body. At first, he wasn't hungry every three hours, so I asked him to start with smaller portions and allow his body—his circadian rhythms, hormones, and metabolism—to recognize the consistent behavior modification. This reduced the pressure his body was carrying. We changed his workouts as well, moving them to the morning (since switching to a morning workout has many brain benefits such as "improved decision-making skills and memory"[35]) and starting with walks, yoga, and Pilates until his body felt energized for more. When your body is ready for more, you know you are reducing your stress level. Some of those signs are being more alert, feeling stronger, and wanting to exercise more.

It was difficult at first, but in two months we were able to make some progress. Now, when he wakes up, he gets his body into sunlight first thing in the morning because this tells his brain that it's time to wake up. He then starts moving his body with a quick five-minute HIIT class. It sounds simple, but it helps to reset his circadian rhythm while lowering his stress hormones.

Jake's sleep issues made him feel inadequate and ashamed, like he was a failure. The reality is that his sleep issues were his body's physical reaction to stress. He was not at fault for his sleep issues, but he could course-correct them. And you're not at fault for any sleep issues you may have.

Not being able to fall asleep or stay asleep is worth a conversation with your primary physician to look at what is going on to cause this dysregulation. You should make it a priority to put your body back in balance, as it will improve your overall well-being and health.

✳ 17 ✳

GET SEVEN HOURS OF SLEEP—YOU UP?

Sometimes we've just grown so used to being tired and sluggish that we don't connect it back to a lack of sleep or realize how important sleep is to our overall health. Our bodies thrive on consistency: they love to wake up at the same time every day, poop at the same time, eat the same amount of food from one day to the next, and fall asleep around the same time. When we develop a routine, our body has less stress and metabolic dysregulation is a thing of the past. Of course, there will be times when we get a bit off, but we have to work on the way we react so we can quickly recover and help our body reach its peak state of balance. Even if you wake up in the middle of the night tomorrow because your dog ate something that gave him a sour stomach, you still have a choice in how you respond. You can say, "Screw it; I will start again next week"—or you can immediately return to the rules. The choice is yours and always has been. I say

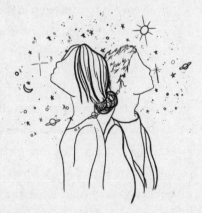

the sooner you get back on a routine, the better. The time you go to sleep and the time you wake up sets the tone for how well your body will function.

In general, there are three main problems you may experience when it comes to sleep:

Problem #1: You can't fall asleep. This is called sleep latency. This often results from having no real sleep schedule, too much caffeine, stress, exercising late in the day, and having too much light exposure before bed.

Problem #2: You can't stay asleep. This often results from anxiety, depression, blood sugar changes, emotional stress, grief, trauma, or worry. It can also be because your room is too warm, or you're exposed to too much light or too much noise, or you have to get up to pee too often throughout the night. The problem is that when you wake up in the middle of the night, your mind switches from sleep mode to wake mode. Your heart rate can increase, your mind can race, and your blood pressure can go up, making it that much harder to go back to sleep. Unfortunately, this is a normal response to stress. The best thing to do is nothing. Don't react, don't count the hours until you are supposed to wake up, and don't take a sleeping aid. Don't sleep in and don't go to bed earlier—just let it go. We can't make up for this lack of sleep; we are better off getting into a structured daily routine. If this problem becomes more chronic, you have some adjustments to make—and I will help you with those in the next chapter.

Problem #3: You wake up in the morning not feeling rested. This is often an issue associated with disruptions in your natural sleep cycles: sleep loss or too much sleep—even naps longer than thirty minutes.[1] The ideal nap time lasts ten to twenty minutes.[2]

Any of these problems can lead to sleep inertia, which is the state between waking and sleep that can lead to disorientation, drowsiness, impaired performance, and a strong desire to go back to sleep. It can last fifteen minutes, an hour, or more. It might make you intoxicated, confused, and slow. You may be experiencing sleep inertia because you are sleep deprived from jet lag or late nights, you're oversleeping or hitting the snooze button, and/or your body just needs more quality sleep. Waking up this way can feel weird—it's like you woke up in the middle of a good night's sleep. Spend some time figuring out what might be going on with your sleep so you can improve its quality.

Here are three of the most common sleep disorders that can cause these sleep symptoms.

1. **Insomnia:** Short-term or long-term, and often linked to other health issues, insomnia is the recurring difficulty in falling asleep and staying asleep. It can be caused by stress, environment, medications, illness, mental health issues, and poor sleep patterns that can cause fatigue, mood swings, and susceptibility to other health problems. Treatment varies, but for chronic conditions, doctors often turn to behavioral therapy.[3]

2. **Sleep apnea:** This is a serious condition in which breathing can actually stop and start during sleep. Loud snoring, gasping for air, and waking with a dry mouth or a sore throat are all possible symptoms. Poor health, being overweight, excessive alcohol consumption, and smoking can put you more at risk. Depending on the severity, treatment can vary from simple lifestyle changes to certain devices that can help open up your airways while you sleep.[4]

3. **Nocturia:** The need to wake up throughout the night to urinate, nocturia is often caused by an overactive bladder. It can be the result of drinking too many fluids, diabetes, fluid retention, certain drugs, and bladder issues. It's often treated by making lifestyle changes (such as restricting fluids) and through medication.[5]

You never want to self-diagnose, so if you feel that you have a sleep disorder, it's in your best interest to be examined by a doctor who can better identify the cause and treat your particular issue.

Maybe you thought, *This is just how I am*—but it doesn't have to be this way. Besides not being able to fall asleep, stay asleep, or wake with energy, you might find that you have extreme fatigue during the day, your sheets are pulled off your bed in the morning, or you have a ton of movement during your sleep. All of these are signs that you might simply need a routine.

If you struggle to sleep at night and don't understand why, you aren't alone. Seventy percent of Americans have reported sleep issues.[6] If you have trouble sleeping, don't automatically assume that you have a disorder, because there are a number of things going on that could impact your sleep:

Certain medications: Some medications can interfere with sleep by causing jitteriness, restlessness, or anxiety. If you are taking a medication, check with your doctor or pharmacist to understand the side effects and what you can do to change them.

Alcohol consumption: How much alcohol do you drink? Alcohol causes the mucus membrane of the nose to thicken, which makes it hard to breathe, so even if you fall asleep, you might have trouble staying asleep. Alcohol interferes with the body's ability to regulate sleep.[7]

Stress: Stress and worry can raise your cortisol levels and make it difficult to sleep.

Sensitivity to noise: Nighttime noise, or, in other words, "unwanted sound," may cause extra production of adrenaline and cortisol as well as increase your heart rate and blood pressure.[8] This will impact your sleep quality and the way you feel the next day.

Sensitivity to light: Exposure to light delays the sleep-promoting hormone, melatonin, from being excreted. Research shows participants exposed to light while sleeping slept ten minutes less per night. This led to confusion during the night, excessive sleepiness, and impaired functioning during the day—overall, it led to more fatigue.[9]

Food sensitivities: I've known patients to get better sleep simply by eliminating their food sensitivities and repairing their gut. The type of sensitivity doesn't particularly matter, but when you have inflammation and don't feel great, your body is stressed, which causes a spike in cortisol.

Overactive bladder or enlarged prostate: Many people tell me they can't sleep because they have to pee multiple times throughout the night.

You can train yourself not to get up during the night: start by not drinking any fluids after 6 PM. Avoid caffeine, carbonated drinks, and alcohol. Empty your bladder before bed.

No matter which problem you suffer from, the first thing to do is develop healthy habits that will lead to getting a better night's sleep. Good sleep is not always easy, but it's worth working on. Sleep is a fundamental pillar in good health. When you have good sleep habits, your body runs the way it should.

✴ 18 ✴

GET SEVEN HOURS OF SLEEP—A GUIDE TO SLEEPING WELL

Lack of sleep can wreak havoc on almost every part of your life and your health, but by getting seven hours of sleep a night you can improve so many different issues. It doesn't seem simple when you're suffering, but it's probably a lot easier to fix the problem than you think. You are so much more in control of your sleep than you realize. There are a number of things you can start doing immediately to help you get better sleep at night so you wake up feeling rested.

The most important thing is to get on a consistent sleep schedule. I've talked about this a lot because it's so vital! It also means no napping throughout the day. Melatonin levels follow your circadian rhythm, so they love a good habit. The best habit you can get into is going to bed and waking up at the same time every day to create a natural circadian rhythm.

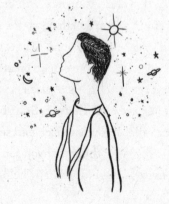

Never hit the snooze button and go back to sleep. Hitting the snooze button is telling your body to fall back into another sleep cycle, which can make you disoriented and groggy, extending sleepiness for two to four hours into the morning.[1] Instead, when you get up in the morning, go out in the sunlight, which tells your body that it's time to wake up. Try to get out in the sunlight every day if possible. As we discussed earlier, our body's clock responds to light as the signal to wake up and dark as the signal to go to sleep. If you have trouble waking up in the morning, finding the sun or even a sun lamp can have dramatic effects on your energy and wake–sleep cycle, because exposure to light in the morning causes nighttime melatonin production to occur sooner, allowing you to sleep more easily at night.[2] If you can get in the habit of taking a walk outside (cloudy or clear) at the same time every day, you will notice your daytime cognitive function, decision-making, and energy levels improve.[3] (And if you can't get outside, you can try simply smelling coffee in the morning, even if you don't drink it: this alerts your mind it's time to wake up.[4])

Make dates with friends to go for walks early in the morning to give you a reason to get moving outside. If you want to take this up a notch, find a way to create consequences for canceling, which will ensure that you follow through and create a new healthy habit.

I'd also recommend that you develop a morning routine in general, because our bodies rely on rhythm. That doesn't mean you have to create a new routine from scratch. Look for ways to make your regular routine more relaxing. So after you wash your face and brush your teeth in the morning, you can apply lavender and aromatherapy, for example. Put your workout clothes on before you leave your bedroom. Plan to head right out the door as soon as you can. It's been proven that five deep breaths can relax your nervous system, and when it comes to getting better sleep, so much of it comes down to the nervous system. So just breathe! That's it. Start by taking five deep breaths, the type of breath that inflates your stomach and sends oxygen to every part of your body.

The other thing that you can do throughout the day to help you sleep better at night is laugh. It actually helps. When you experience stress for long periods of time, your body becomes very tense. Laughter produces endorphins that help relieve pain and relax your nervous system.

Make sure you're following the rules and getting in your 10,000 steps throughout the day, because moving your body will reduce cortisol levels. Walking, yoga, and Pilates are all great forms of exercise that help improve your sleep and cortisol levels. When researchers compared sedentary but otherwise healthy older adults over the age of sixty who they then placed in different forms of activity, participants who complained of sleep disturbances over a two-and-a-half-year period who did low-impact exercises had greater improvements in sleep overall.[5] In another twelve-month study, participants engaged in home-based exercise outdoors found a positive impact on sleep quality, felt more rested, and fell asleep quicker.[6]

You should also try to cut back on caffeine and alcohol. In fact, try to eliminate caffeine in the evening. Too much caffeine in the evening can keep you up. You don't want to fall into the vicious cycle of drinking too much coffee because you are groggy from not sleeping. All you're doing is jacking up all of your stress hormones and making the problem worse. And, just like caffeine, alcohol can have a severe impact on your ability to fall asleep, stay asleep, and get good quality sleep, so if you're trying to get on a healthy sleep schedule, eliminate caffeine and alcohol as best you can. And as I've mentioned, cutting back on your water intake in the evening will help prevent the need to get up to use the restroom. If you find yourself frequently getting up to pee in the middle of the night, try to finish drinking most of your water about three to four hours before you go to sleep.

Eating too much at night can keep you up and make it difficult to fall asleep. You will sleep better if you try to avoid eating four to six hours before your bedtime.[7] When we eat, our body works to digest, absorb, and metabolize food. If that happens at night, it's stopping our bodies from resting, as one study found: "Eating or drinking less than one hour before bedtime is associated with increased risk of wake after sleep onset."[8] Sometimes we need a small snack, because on occasion we are too hungry to go to sleep.[9] After all, being too hungry can make it hard to fall asleep, too, so in these cases, eat a *small* snack, and give your body fifteen minutes—you'll probably find it was all you needed until the morning.

Remember to be structured in the rules and flexible with how they play out. There will be nights when you need something to eat because maybe you just didn't eat enough during the day. And this is okay; one day is no big deal. Two days in a row could be habit forming, which we are trying to prevent. So be thoughtful during the day. However, please don't restrict during the day in an attempt to make up for whatever happens at night. Hopefully, after getting to this point in the book, you see why it's so important to balance our blood sugar and to eat small meals throughout the day to prevent just this kind of thing from happening. But I still want to explicitly say that even if you did eat the night before, you can and should still eat throughout the day. Get yourself back into the rhythm of consistency.

Nighttime is when many people feel entitled to eat or are looking for a "treat." We have trained ourselves to think that having something sweet after dinner or before going to bed is our reward after a full day of work. Every day I hear people justify late-night eating with statements like, "I love my chocolate," or "I was good all day," and "It's just one little chocolate."

Do we really need more food after dinner? Maybe sometimes, but absolutely not all the time. Because we are pleasure seekers, maybe at some point in our day we planted a seed that we would be having a drink or eating a bowl of ice cream. Why would we deny ourselves something delicious; don't we deserve it? But we have done it so many times that it's become an automatic habit. I urge you to consult the Wellness Wheel and figure out where to find connection rather than seeking it from food. If you are hungry, then eat, absolutely! But that shouldn't be an everyday thing—and if you're eating because you're feeling something other than hunger, it shouldn't be an *any* day thing. If you want ice cream, eat ice cream during the day when you are hungry. And use your me time instead as a chance to use the Wellness Wheel to connect to what you need. Because I am afraid eating ice cream or pretzels at 9 PM is exactly the opposite of taking care of our needs. It's time to rethink the way we love ourselves.

Here are the facts: nobody is *always* hungry after dinner. Instead, you are giving in to what you are feeling—fear, anxiety, entitlement, or a search for fun and a source of comfort—which is a bad habit that needs to be broken. And if you do experience physical hunger in the evening, it means you are not eating enough during the day, so you need to change how much you eat throughout the day.

I had a client tell me that he never felt hungry in the morning. After talking some more, I learned that he always snacked in the afternoon, which was his family's culture. The snacks continued late into the evening, and he felt out of control. So we flipped his eating schedule and spaced out his meals. And like clockwork, he started losing weight and regulating his blood sugars, and ended the evening binges. We both cheered when he started getting hungry in the morning; it meant that his metabolism was boosted and he could use that food as fuel and not as comfort, fun, or a reward. It meant that food would no longer be stored as fat. Making this simple change helped him lose weight and keep it off.

You need to do the same thing—let your body regulate. And focus on a routine. We are not striving for perfection but looking to regularly make strides. This focus will allow you to be curious about how and when to make some adjustments. When your body's clock is out of sync, you feel off and make poor choices. It doesn't matter if you are a nurse who works nights or someone who travels abroad every month—it's important to get yourself into a consistent routine. Your body will respond to the messages you give it. You don't have to know ahead of time what you are eating, or how you will get the steps—just be the person who is intentional in following the six simple rules wherever you are.

One thing to do is to create a relaxing environment. You might drink tea (without caffeine) and dim the lights in your house because that sense of calm will allow your melatonin to naturally rise and get your body in a relaxed state, so you can wind down. If that doesn't do the trick, try taking a warm bath. Or consider starting a meditation practice that includes positive affirmations and mantras before bed. Not only can it help you relax, but you will be training your brain to be more positive.

As briefly mentioned earlier, alcohol and sleep don't mix well. Alcohol should not be used as a sleep aid. Alcohol initially acts as a sedative, so we can fall asleep faster—but there is much evidence that alcohol becomes activating as it's metabolized, "resulting in fragmented and disturbed sleep in the second half of the night."[10] Plus, when you drink consistently, your body develops a tolerance for the sedating effects and you are left with wakefulness.[11] Drinking alcohol in moderation is generally considered safe, but each one of us will react differently and need to pay attention to what our body needs. Think of it this way: a serving or a drink is considered twelve ounces of beer, one ounce of liquor, or five ounces of wine. "Low" levels of drinking are less than two drinks for men and less than one drink for women; even this level, though, was found to decrease sleep quality by 9.3 percent. Moderate drinking is classified as approximately two drinks for a man and one drink for a woman—and is linked to a 24 percent dip in sleep quality. Men who drink more than two drinks and women who drink more than one drink are considered to be heavier drinkers—and that's a level that's been shown to reduce sleep quality by 39.2 percent.[12] So don't turn to alcohol as a sleep aid—it may be detrimental to your sleep.

Another thing that you can do to become a better sleeper is to set your bedroom temperature to cool. When you sleep your body temperature drops, so sleeping in a cooler room will help your temperature drop faster; keeping your body at that lower temperature will help you stay asleep as well. Light of any kind can suppress melatonin secretion and delay sleep,[13] and our electronics actually emit a blue light that is also a suppressor. To encourage melatonin production, avoid looking at bright screens a few hours before bed and expose yourself to bright lights during the day. If you absolutely have to look at a screen before bed, try wearing blue light glasses. And definitely avoid work emails, social media, the news, or anything else that can cause you stress and raise your cortisol levels before you go to sleep. Get in the habit of saying no to what causes you and your body stress.

By far, the biggest mistake that you can make when readjusting your sleep habits is to quit just when you're starting the process because you don't see immediate results. If you start going to sleep at the same time every night, and waking up at the same time every morning, you aren't suddenly going to feel great the first day, or even the second day. It will take time to reset your body clock and your circadian rhythm. How much time it takes depends on the person and their circumstances, but if you do it every day for weeks and months, your body *will* adjust, and it *will* become natural.

It all goes back to resetting your wellness compass. Until you do, it's so easy to slip back into old patterns when you experience triggers, encounter resistance, or just don't see results. When your alarm goes off in the morning and you're still exhausted, it's so easy to say, "Screw it," and go back to sleep. You are rationalizing a bad idea—but that's what happens when you're tired. That's why, no matter how hard it is out of the gate, stick with it, and create a routine. You'll see the results—trust me!

All of these rules take practice. Think of it this way: I've had clients who have lost forty pounds, but for the first couple of weeks, they didn't lose anything. For some of them, it took a month before they saw any results at all. Why? Because if you've had the same habits and been at the same weight for years and decades, your body might need more time to adjust. While it might be hard to be patient when you're struggling to see results or feel that you can't make the changes necessary to get enough healthy, natural sleep, try your best to not turn to the pharmacy counter. I believe it's best to do things naturally to achieve positive sustainable change when it comes to sleep. And if you come to rely on sleep aids, convincing yourself that you need them to sleep well, you are doing yourself a disservice in the long run when it comes to getting natural healthy sleep. There may be circumstances and issues that require medication, but you want to try making changes before you resort to taking something to sleep.

When you know why you are having trouble falling asleep or staying asleep, you can get the right support your body needs to heal.

YOU ARE IN CONTROL

Do you want to wake up and feel good in the morning? Do you want to be energized throughout the day, and not feel sluggish or like you have to take a nap? When it finally clicks, and you fall into a rhythm that allows you to get enough sleep, everything starts to flow smoothly. To reach this goal, you need to prioritize your sleeping habits.

We all need consistent quality sleep. If you aren't sleeping, you need to figure out why. This is a nut that has to be cracked. You don't want to do all of this work when it comes to food and exercise only to have your progress limited because you aren't sleeping well at night.

The good news is that just as easily as you trained yourself to be a poor sleeper, you can course-correct and learn how to sleep well once again. Take a closer look at your behaviors and try to pinpoint the problem. If you can't get to the bottom of it, turn to a professional who might be able to help find natural ways to put your body back into homeostasis. It doesn't have to be your primary care physician; ask for a referral or find a specialist. And during your visit, make sure you bring a list of concerns and stay on track. Make sure you get an explanation for what is happening and don't settle for generic excuses or medications. You might not like the answers you get, but learning what you don't know is empowering, and there is always more you can do.

I believe almost every sleep-related problem can be improved by making lifestyle changes, so the ball is in your court.

✳ THE RULE #6
WRAP-UP

We need sleep! Sleep affects everything from how we feel to how we make choices in our day to how well our body functions. The average adult does not get enough sleep; we need to aim for seven hours each night and change the average. Our health is vital, and good sleep habits need to be a priority, so what can you do today to improve your sleep health?

Set a consistent sleep schedule: go to sleep at the same time and wake at the same time.
Move your body daily, preferably in the sunlight.
Limit your naps to twenty minutes or less.

Notice if alcohol is affecting your sleep.

Consider what you are eating before bed, and make sure you are hungry or put it on hold until tomorrow. You will probably not remember what you ate, but lack of sleep will wreak havoc in your day and body.

Remind your subconscious you are a good sleeper.

Trust that you can change and *will* change with consistency.

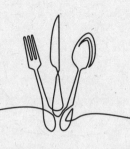

PUTTING IT ALL TOGETHER

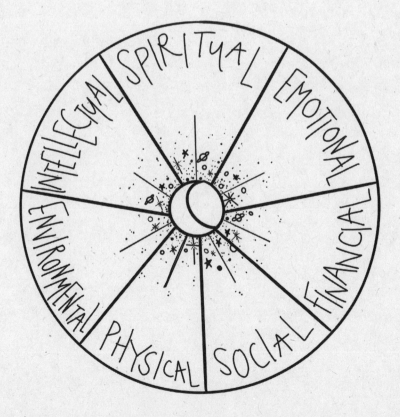

✳ 19 ✳

PUTTING IT ALL TOGETHER—FREE WILL

"If this illness feels right now like a cage, please try to hear me: it isn't locked. It has been open all along. You are free to go."

I often share this quote by Marya Hornbacher with my clients, replacing the word "illness" with "disordered eating." Because while you've been trapped in your bad habits, you are free to change them. By following these six rules, you are allowing yourself to be free. Yes, the wider world can be scary—but can you get curious and see what happens? Can you trust yourself?

After all these years I understand why people stay stuck: it comes down to comfort in their discomfort. They know exactly how this goes and how it feels to be stuck, and to walk out of the cage they made themselves comfortable in is really, really scary. People don't walk willingly into fear. Especially if they have failed so many times. But the choice to walk out and to recognize you have survived every single moment and that you are capable of taking care of yourself because you are worth it is how you build both trust and confidence.

HOW DO YOU SHOW UP IN THE WORLD?

We all walk around carrying a load of labels. It's how we show up in the world, how people think of us, and how we think of ourselves. Ego-based thinking, these labels make us try to fit into them—and when we don't, they leave us with guilt and shame. How do you label yourself? Here are some of mine:

- Mom
- Wife
- Daughter
- Sister
- Dietitian
- Non-dieter
- Normal Eater
- Anxious
- Joyful
- Athlete (sort of)
- Migraine Sufferer
- Peaceful
- Overwhelmed
- Empath
- Friend
- Teacher
- Healer
- Author

I could come up with dozens, but you get the idea. Take a pen and a piece of paper and start jotting down all of the different ways in which you regularly show up in the world.

Even though we have a list of who we are and what makes us unique, we are so much more. Maybe your list included Dieter, Failed Dieter, Overweight, Sad, Stress Eater, Lazy, Lonely. It doesn't matter. I want you to make another list and title it "Who am I without these labels?" There is only one answer: anything you want to be. What would it be like if you could say no and not worry about another person's reaction? What would it be like for you to not feel the need to please people?

From now on, I want you to think of yourself not as a label but someone free of labels—be anything you want. Be anything and be everything. Especially when it comes to food and the way you eat, if you are looking for a sustainable change you must let go of who you think you are. Remember the cage—the door is open. Labels will hold you back.

TAKING ACTION

You have the power to be whoever you want. In fact, you have more power than you realize. Use your power wisely. Remember, it doesn't matter what anyone else is doing or eating. You can eat meat or fish for lunch; you can choose vegetarian; it doesn't matter. You don't have to label your eating. Eat what you want, and do it without judgment. But do it with love and be kind to your body, eat when you are hungry, and eat foods that make you feel great.

Today, do this: be flexible with what you eat; just follow the six rules.

✎ What happens when you eat when you are hungry?

_____

_____

✎ What happens when you eat what you love?

_____

_____

Now repeat this at your next meal.

I have a client who told me right out of the gate that she was a binge eater. What she didn't realize was that she brings that mentality into every food situation. So if she were to walk into the kitchen and see a bowl of blueberries, she could easily rationalize eating more of them because they're "healthy" and she tells herself that she's a binge eater. It has nothing to do with whether she's hungry or not. She's become attached to that label, so we must sever that cord. She can be the type of eater that scans her body and honors what she needs moment to moment.

Another way we can label ourselves is with schedules and routines. I have so many clients tell me things like, "I eat lunch at noon," or "I need to have vegetables with that meal." Why? Who says that? If I woke up at 6 AM, why would I have to wait until noon to eat lunch? Who knows how I will feel any given day at noon? Sometimes I work out before lunch, and sometimes I work out after. That can change my level of hunger. You might have eaten a bowl of fruit last night after dinner. That doesn't mean you have to eat it tonight. You might want it tomorrow, but you don't need to decide now.

Being a normal eater is detaching yourself from your labels. Instead, live in this moment. I'm not telling you to neglect your responsibilities or offend other people. I am telling you to drop the labels when it comes to food and give yourself permission to be whatever you want. If you didn't have to live with all those labels you jotted down on the page, who would you be at this moment? Forget your ego and get in touch with your authentic self. Only eat when you are hungry and eat what you love without fear or judgment. You can have more if you're still hungry, or you can get up and walk away from the table even if you aren't completely satisfied because you know that you will eat again.

Labels are dangerous. They make it hard to branch out. Watch how you view food and drop the labels.

Take my client Lexie, for example: At the beginning of our session she told me how she was really good at eating half unless she let herself get too hungry. Then she went on to say she couldn't control herself around "gross" foods like mac and cheese. But the truth is most people can't control themselves when they get that hungry. So practice not getting to the point of starving—but also, if you like it, it's not "gross." I love mac and cheese; it's an anytime food for me, just not something at the top of my list. If I thought I couldn't have it, I might want it more.

My solution with Lexie was for her to begin noticing how she referred to food, and to give herself permission to eat food, any food, all food. Instead of labeling the food or letting herself get too hungry, she could take it slow by scanning her body, by knowing what she was feeling, by eating what she loved so she was making more self-controlled decisions that felt empowered.

Another example is my client Sam, who started our conversation by telling me, "I know I need to take care of myself and stop eating pizza, pasta, and beef." He also told me he struggles with eating half. But most people would when they are restricting themselves and labeling food like he was. Sam was trying to eat "healthy" foods and then seeking what he really wanted after. Sam needed to get out of his own way; he needed to learn that he could have these foods and still lose weight. He needed to see he was in control. When he was empowered to eat what he loved and when he recognized how the foods he loved made him feel, he could then try other things. There are no bad foods unless it makes you sick. So when he—or you—eats what he loves and starts with half, he won't have the need to overeat because he knows he can have more later.

And then we have Janna. Janna was known around town and in her family as a dieter. She loved this title and felt pride in knowing the latest and greatest diets. Janna is seventy-five years old and sixty pounds overweight, and she suffers from high blood pressure, high blood sugar, high triglycerides, high cholesterol—metabolic syndrome. Her doctors had prescribed her medications for all these ailments, but she was taking all this medication at night with water, so it was causing her to wake up multiple times to use the restroom, which disrupted her sleep. She also had to repair her gut, because there are forty-five foods that she is sensitive to—these were causing inflammation, so she clears her throat and wipes her runny nose all day.

Janna has been on countless diets, and usually loses weight on all of them, but she can't keep the weight off, which is the source of so many of her health issues. Every time she lost weight, she gained back more, laughing it off, promising herself and everyone else she would be losing it again soon enough. When she started working with me and following the six rules, she had never done anything like it before in her life, but she was dedicated to being an A student. She lost ten pounds in the first two and a half weeks. Not only is she now walking four miles a day, and waking up only once during the night, but when her husband recently made her lunch, she only ate half because she realized she wasn't hungry. At this rate, she will be decreasing her medication very soon. More importantly, she's learned how to keep the weight off. Labels can keep us stuck; without labels we can be anything we want. Now Janna is simply someone who eats when she is hungry and eats what she wants. And what's more is that she is lowering some of her meds and discontinuing some others. Go, Janna!

Don't expect change to happen right away. I mean, it could: most of my clients tell me by their second appointment they had no idea how easy it is. But it can also take time. Think of this like you're in training, and it all starts with being intentional. There will be people who have certain opinions when they see you eating what you love, but ignore those opinions. Drop the labels and ignore what others think they know. No one can do this for you. There will be days when it's effortless, and there will be days when you need to put intention into every move you make. There will be moments when your mind will give you an excuse or rationalize a decision that you know is not aligned with your wellness compass and not in your best interest. When you encounter that resistance, find grace within yourself, understand we are only human, and go back to the rules. This is life, and successful people keep going. That's how you heal your wellness compass. The only way you can mess this up is by giving up.

✳ 20 ✳

PUTTING IT ALL TOGETHER—PROGRESS OVER PERFECTION

There will always be a new fad diet around the corner, and there will always be people who fall for them. Those diets might even help a few people lose weight, but the odds are stacked against you if your goal is to keep the weight off. Don't get distracted by the shiny new objects. Keep your eye on the prize.

Today is a new day. This moment is a new moment. Choose you every time. Go back and re-read your *why*. I want to remind you that your first actual achievement is the moment you choose to keep going, even when it's easier to give up. And it's so easy to give up. It's so easy to start tomorrow. Don't do it. Don't think short term; don't plan on failing; take it one day at a time. One moment at a time.

Winning does not come from losing weight; winning comes from keeping the weight off. Learn to develop your strengths from your struggles because the struggles will pass. Practice standing still and allowing yourself to feel stress, discomfort, boredom, fear—you have everything you need inside of you to survive these moments. If you are good at keeping promises to others, make that same commitment to yourself. The cost of being unwell is so high: bad choices increase your mental and physical stress leading to both anxiety and depression. Being well is worth it—you are worth it. No matter how unbalanced you feel, it is possible to rebalance with consistency and practice.

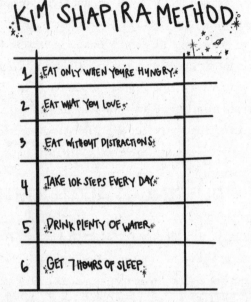

KIM SHAPIRA METHOD

1. EAT ONLY WHEN YOU'RE HUNGRY.
2. EAT WHAT YOU LOVE.
3. EAT WITHOUT DISTRACTIONS.
4. TAKE 10K STEPS EVERY DAY.
5. DRINK PLENTY OF WATER.
6. GET 7 HOURS OF SLEEP.

Pretty soon, you will realize that your *why* becomes the process itself. You made it up to the top of the hill, backpack full of rocks and all. Some moments were tough—maybe you even stopped a few times along the way, or got lost and had to change course—but you kept going. You encountered bad weather, sore muscles, and numerous distractions, but you kept moving and realized that it wasn't that difficult anymore. You practiced transitioning from one moment to the next while remaining unaffected. You practiced a new way of thinking and acting—a way where one bad meeting didn't cause you to spiral until you could get home and soothe yourself with a "treat."

The backpack felt lighter, and, once you reached the top, you realized that you didn't require a family member in need as a source of motivation. You did it all on your own, and that's empowering. Now you know that it can be done and are confident that you can do it again. That's exhilarating! More significantly, you learned to love and appreciate the journey that you're on now.

If you follow all six rules simultaneously, you will continue to see results. Your weight might fluctuate because of factors such as salt and hormones, but you should not plateau until you get to your normal weight for your body. Eating only what your body needs will help you drop weight. The steps will allow your body fat to decrease along with your weight, while the water flushes your system, and the sleep will allow your body to be in balance. Altogether, the process allows you to become a metabolic machine with all six burners on.

If you feel like you are not seeing results or are not losing weight, check in with your Wellness Wheel (see page 40). See what might be driving you to ignore the rules and which areas in your life need more attention. The goal is to get into a routine, which helps to keep your new behaviors in check no matter what else (from a vacation to a deadline, to a holiday or a stressful situation) might be happening in your life. Are you following the rules, or have you slipped back into old habits and beliefs? It doesn't really matter why you slipped; it's more important to realize you slipped and get right back to valuing your why.

I know you're thinking that this all sounds good in theory, but it will get tougher when real life sets in. Real life involves holidays, vacations, anniversaries, parties, deadlines, sick kids, pandemics, and sleepless nights. But the rules fit in with real life, I promise. Especially because what matters is *progress* and not perfection. So plan on taking this new lifestyle mentality and the six simple rules with you everywhere life takes you. If you overeat one night, don't allow it to derail you and don't beat yourself up. Get back on track. Don't strive for perfection. Just hold yourself accountable. Reach out to a friend if necessary. You don't need to do this alone.

KEEPING YOURSELF ACCOUNTABLE

An old client of mine whom I hadn't seen in fifteen years recently returned to one of my groups. It was great to see her again, but it was a reminder of how much my method had changed over the years because it was her first time seeing these rules. During her first week back, she did something interesting. She broke down each rule, gave herself a letter grade for the week, and then came up with her cumulative score for each rule and a total for all six. This shed light on areas where she needed work, and it allowed her to better set her intentions going forward. She could then compare her GPA week to week, or even day to day if she wanted to. I liked this so much that I adopted it and encouraged my other clients to do the same.

As you master the rules, it's important to set aside time each week to evaluate your progress and identify the areas that are challenging you. Use this time to recenter yourself and set new mini goals. Report cards are graded by you for you. They exist to spark conversation with yourself, which will allow you to be your own growth partner. The report cards are not a weapon; they are not meant to be used for self-abuse.

You're doing your best! Imagine you are grading your best friend's progress, or your child's progress. Treat yourself as you would treat your favorite person in the world. If you wouldn't say it to them, don't say it to yourself.

Every week, rate yourself on how well you followed each rule from 0 to 100 percent. Then add up each of your scores and divide by five to find your average for the week based on the following scale:

90 to 100 percent: Get it!
Yes! You're killing it. My educated guess is you lost weight, gained confidence, and are running on diesel-level inner power.

80 to 89 percent: Celebrate your wins!
Maybe you forgot to drink water this weekend or you restricted your food during some meals. That's okay! You're definitely putting in the effort. Make a note of where you can improve and celebrate the things you did well!

70 to 79 percent: Keep going!
If you didn't lose any weight, don't get frustrated. Reflect on the moments you feel you could improve. Where were you? What were your triggers? How were you feeling? How can you avoid a similar situation this week? Give yourself praise for the moments you succeeded, and push through the discomfort because that is the formula for growth.

69 percent and lower: Make a game plan!
Things didn't go the way you wished they had. That's okay. Like all relationships, your relationship with food will have its ups and downs. Instead of being discouraged, make a new game plan to improve. Use your failures as fuel. Flip the script.

I have an eighteen-year-old client who had gone from one hundred and sixty to two hundred pounds in the two years before he first came to see me.

I wasn't able to fit him in for three weeks, but I told him to keep detailed food records prior to our first meeting. Over the next three weeks, he ate two meals a day and walked an average of 2,300 steps a day. He showed up to our first appointment weighing the exact same as he weighed when we spoke—two hundred pounds.

I explained the six rules, and after the first week, he had a grade of 90 percent and lost eight and a half pounds. Over the next three months, he bounced between 80 and 90 percent and lost twenty-five pounds, all while traveling all over the world. He has learned the power of the rules, seeing how his body responds, so now that he is headed off to college, he plans to maintain that B average and follow the rules 80 percent of the time, so he can continue to see results.

Today, I can say without a doubt that this works. Every single time I do a follow-up appointment, I go through each rule and ask the client to grade themselves. I've learned that if they have an A or above, following the rules 90 percent of the time, they are losing between three and five pounds per week. A B average (80 percent) translates to about one half pound to a full pound per week. If they're only following the rules 70 percent of the time, they're learning a bunch of new techniques but aren't losing weight. And at 60 percent and below, they're typically gaining weight.

Alternatively, if the gray areas in that scoring system feel daunting, you can also simply mark how many days you followed a rule to give yourself a weekly score out of seven. In other words, if you followed Rule #6 for five out of seven days, you'd have a 5 for that rule. You'd add that to your scores for the other rules (and your maximum, 7+7+7+7+7+7, would be 42) and divide that number by 6 (because there are six rules). That would give you your average score for the week. As you continue to evaluate yourself, you'll start to see what average you need to be at to keep meeting your goals.

While you can use your phone or an Apple Watch to check your steps, there is very little you can do to precisely chart your progress with some of the other rules. So the scoring system can help fill that void. Scoring may not work for everyone, but give it a shot and see if it helps you.

Alternatively, you might just like a habit tracker like this:

	M	T	W	T	F	S	S
Rule #1 Eat When I am Hungry: breakfast (B)							
*Start with Half (B)							
Rule #2 Eat What I Love (B)							
Rule #3 Eat Without Distractions (B)							
Rule #1 Eat When I am Hungry: snack (S)							
*Start with Half (S)							
Rule #2 Eat What I Love (S)							
Rule #3 Eat Without Distractions (S)							
Rule #1 Eat When I am Hungry: lunch (L)							
*Start with Half (L)							
Rule #2 Eat What I Love (L)							
Rule #3 Eat Without Distractions (L)							
Rule #1 Eat When I am Hungry: snack (S)							
*Start with Half (S)							
Rule #2 Eat What I Love (S)							
Rule #3 Eat Without Distractions (S)							
Rule #1 Eat When I am Hungry: dinner (D)							
*Start with Half (D)							
Rule #2 Eat What I Love (D)							
Rule #3 Eat Without Distractions (D)							
Rule #4 Get 10,000 Steps							
Rule #5 Drink Eight Cups of Water							
Rule #6 Get Seven Hours of Sleep							

A Word of Warning

Sheila was heartbroken because her family desperately wanted her to lose weight. When I first met with her, she had a history of binge eating and she was very sedentary. She felt a lot of shame when it came to food, so much so that for the first few months we met, she could never look me in the eye, and we rarely ever talked about food. She struggled with the first three rules, but she excelled when it came to getting in her steps.

Sheila went from being completely sedentary to walking 30,000 steps every day. She would get up early and go on a five- to ten-mile hike. When she'd go to business meetings around town, she would make sure to park blocks away from the restaurant or office. It worked! She lost fifty pounds, and I was so proud because I could tell how much it meant to her. However, it breaks my heart to say that she is not a success story, because she was never able to work on the food component. She could not apply the first three rules, so guess what happened? She couldn't keep the weight off.

This example reiterates why you need to use all of the rules. When you try to cut corners and think you can do it on just one or two rules, you will fail. It's critical that you incorporate all of them into your lifestyle to be successful. Trust me, I have seen what happens when you do not.

So whenever you feel like your grades just aren't matching up to your goals, remember to go back to the Wellness Wheel to examine all of the spokes on that wheel. Those spokes represent places in your life that might be impacting the choices that you make. In other words, examining the spokes can help you get curious about your habits—and about how you can change those habits so that you can find fulfillment in things that aren't edible.

The choices we make every day are made from one of two places:

1. Trust: I am safe. I know I have enough. There will be more later. I can have fun without a drink or eating when I am not hungry.
2. Fear: Everyone else is doing it. I don't want to miss out. I will start tomorrow. I am uncomfortable making different food choices than those around me.

Unfortunately, we often operate from a place of fear because we are hard-wired to survive. If you feel deprived, you immediately think you want it and must have it. It's our natural default. If everyone is sitting around eating tacos, and you know that you can't eat tacos, will the peer pressure or fear of missing out be so much that you give in? If your significant other is up late and wants something to eat, will you feel the need to join? A lot of people do, even though they know what they need. But sometimes saying no is really saying yes to yourself. Eating something to not feel left out, persecuting yourself for eating it, and then feeling ashamed is not an act of self-love.

If you don't love yourself when making choices, you are most likely doing yourself harm. If you love yourself, trust yourself, and take care of yourself, you will treat yourself the way that you would treat someone you love.

Some people will struggle with the food, some with the steps, and some with the water. It won't all be easy right away, but keep at it. Think of every day and every meal as a reset. Strive to make small, gradual changes to improve your daily habits. Find wins, and practice your progress. The goal isn't just weight loss; it's sustainable weight loss, which requires change. If you want that change to stick, you need to enjoy the journey and not only be looking forward to reaching the destination.

This method is about standing in your own truth. It's about not needing to belong to the "in" crowd or thinking about what's "healthy" or "unhealthy." It's about getting and staying well. It's about ignoring what others think and being okay with exactly who you are with food. It's about staying in your own lane and being the leader of your own body. It's about shredding guilt, finding peace, and making it normal to eat the foods you love. It's about loving yourself. The kind of love you actually deserve.

ACKNOWLEDGMENTS

Thanks to my husband, Matt, my biggest supporter and encourager. Thank you for bringing me coffee every morning. Thank you to my daughters Olivia, Sophia, and Natasha for being my greatest gifts and teachers. Your lessons are endless, and I think I have done a pretty good job planting seeds to make you strong, capable humans in a world full of fear around food.

Thank you to my parents, Nancy and David. You two are the absolute best. I appreciate my education and your love and support and guidance more than words can say. Thank you for guiding me to be a teacher in my own way and encouraging me to be more than I thought possible. Thank you to my brother, Matt, for letting me practice "teaching" when we were growing up. I love you and always feel my best when you are in the room with me. Brenda, my big sister, thank you for supporting me and always stepping in when I need you. To my niece, Sydney, and my nephew, Harry, I love you both; thank you for making me an aunt. To my in-laws, Don and Tamara, thank you for your enthusiasm and support. I appreciated all your encouragement and discussions throughout this process.

My agent, Nena Madonia—I am so grateful for you. Nena, the universe put you next to me for a reason, and I hope you stay there forever. The timing of our meeting was and still is profound to me—when I told you that you needed to know me, it was a big step in my personal growth. Thank you for listening to me and believing in me and for getting me here. You are such an incredibly gifted soul sister. You are creative, organized, and quick witted, and I am so happy I get to work with you.

Loan Dang, my rock, my lawyer, my friend—well, you are everything. You could literally manage my whole family and yours, and I thank you from the bottom of my heart for everything. Michael Pelmont, I also thank you for everything. (Although Loan deserves all the credit.)

Thank you to my entire team at BenBella. A special thank-you to my publisher, Glenn Yeffeth, for taking a chance on me. I am forever grateful to my editor, Alyn Wallace, who helped me shape and hone *This Is What You're Really Hungry For.* Alyn, I loved you from our first call. Thank you for taking my first draft and turning it into what it is now. You have an incredible eye, and I thank you for every guiding note and line of feedback. We did it. Elizabeth Degenhard, thank you for all your hard work and your critical eye; both are very appreciated. Sarah Avinger and Brigid Pearson—I love my cover. Thank you for really working hard for this one. It's better than I could have ever dreamed up. To my director of marketing, Lindsay Marshall and Kellie Doherty, thank you both for all of your hard work. Madeline Grigg, I am so grateful to you and all your efforts; thank you. To my deputy publisher Adrienne Lang, thank you. A special thank-you to the vendor content manager, Alicia Kania, and to Sarah Beck for all of your help—it is so appreciated. And thank you to Aida Herrera for all that you do. Rachel Phares, thank you for handling the contract. Kim Broderick, thank you for shepherding my book through the final stages. Lastly, Raquel Moreno, thank you. Writing a book has always been my dream. I appreciate all of you collaborating and communicating with me through this entire process. Your advice and guidance have been invaluable to me. I feel so lucky to be part of your community. To everyone who had their hands on this at BenBella, I so appreciate it. Let's go do great things!

Cynthia Romans, the biggest thank-you for being my at-home, loving caregiver while I was at work or writing. You take great loving care of my family, my dogs, and my house. Thank you for feeding us and for all of your coffee runs. We love you so much.

To my clients—each and every one of you. You have all had as much of an impact on me as I hope I have had on you. I learned what worked and where I needed to do the work. I am stronger and better because of you. Thank you for trusting me with your health, and thank you for your constant encouragement and feedback. We all have our own personal stories playing out, and you all are part of mine.

Jenny Hutt, I think you are so badass on so many levels. Thank you for bringing me on to your show and allowing me the space to help all of your listeners. I am so honored to have been a part of your Weight Wednesday.

My book club: Becky Vitner, Tracy Shaffer, Karine Chung, Autumn Krischer, Fiona Hutton, Bridgette Fischer, Kim Hinton, Rachelle Wells, Andrea Epinger, Galit Shokrian, Maddie Clark, Janelle Werdesheim, Denise Callahan—from day one you all have been so supportive and enthusiastic. Thank you all for your endless encouragement.

A special thank-you to Josh and Jamie Greenberg. There is nothing better in the world than when people connect and support each other. Josh, thank you for helping me see that I could be and do more. Jamie, thank you for pushing me out of my comfort zone. I really like where I've landed.

Eve Rodsky, thank you for paving the way for me, from concept to creation. I am so thankful for your encouragement and for help with titles. It takes a village, and I am happy you are in mine. You are a rock star, and it has been such an honor to watch you become so much more. And I really think we are just beginning to see how you will change the world.

Elaine Sir, you, lady, are so awesome. Not because you were the first person who saw my message so clearly and pushed me to be more vocal, but because of all that you do. Thank you for being that person for me; I am forever grateful.

To my friends who encourage and support me through it all: thank you for providing the energy to get to the finish line.

Lori Burns, you give the best advice. Your strength is contagious; thank you, my friend.

Jen Wasser, your fashion sense is perfection. And your encouragement is so appreciated. I am sure I owe you a call.

Michal Sperling, your strength and ambition feed my strength and ambition.

Leslie and Michael Thorn, thank you for always getting excited for me and encouraging me.

Autumn Krischer, your endless support and belief in me are so appreciated.

Lauri Metrose, you always make me feel like I can do anything. You never doubted me, and this has given me so much strength.

Laura and Glenn Shubb, I love you two and appreciate every moment we get to spend together. Glenn, remember way back when you helped me outline what the Kim Shapira Method would look like? Your brain is amazing. Laura, there isn't enough space to write all the ways in which I love you.

Stacey Carr, thank you for all of your guidance and support.

Holly Shakoor Fleischer, you have such a special place in my heart. Thank you for deeply understanding my message. I feel so lucky to have you in my life.

Kristin Fairweather, you are for sure the wind beneath my wings. If ever I feel like I just can't, you are right there sprinkling fairy dust all over me, reminding me I can. Thank you.

Ashley Podell, I love you, my friend. You are the best hula-hooper and fiercely badass. I am so lucky to have you in my life.

To my Maj girls, Dr. Myah Gittelson, Kim Anish, Gaby Kaplan, and Melissa Burton: every minute playing with you is just pure fun, and I so appreciate you all for the chitchat, the quarters I win from you, and the quarters I will eventually win from you.

Israel friends, you all came into my life and filled up my heart when I didn't even know I needed you. I think of you all like sisters. Thank you for all your love and support.

Valerie Danna, I am grateful for your constant support and motivation. Your guidance, assistance, and expertise throughout this process have been so appreciated.

Marla Sokoloff, thank you for your endless support and constant sense of humor. Every woman should have a friend like you.

Michal Cohen, thank you for always being down to try something new. Wendy and Jeff Kleid, thank you for always being a constant in my life and for believing in me.

Jade Luna, thank you for being such an amazing astrologer. From our first meeting, when I wasn't sure why I was even having a meeting with you, to now. You have opened my mind and heart to know I am exactly where I need to be.

Ryan Dempsey, thank you so much for making this whole thing possible. Look how far I've come. Thank you for your guidance and support. Katie Jensen, thank you for jumping in and helping me navigate this editing process. I could not have done it without you. And a special thank-you to Kelsey Sante for knowing me, and getting me, and coming to my rescue—you are incredible, and so talented. I so appreciate you.

Norman Cousins, Martin and Shirley Leeds, Micheal Vener, Deborah Raffin, and Carrie Wiatt, I am so lucky to have met you. In so many ways, you are my superheroes, each one lighting up something inside of me. This book and where I am today is because I knew you.

Kaley Cuoco, it has been an absolute pleasure being a part of your life. You are a true inspiration, and I have loved watching you grow into the woman you are. We have been in each other's lives for so long. I remember seeing you when Olivia was just three weeks old—it feels like yesterday, and yet we have both grown and changed so much. I am so happy you wrote my Foreword and are part of my book. My heart is full.

Thank you, dear reader, for taking the time to read this book, and for trusting me with your health.

ENDNOTES

NOT ANOTHER DIET BOOK: WHY USE
THE KIM SHAPIRA METHOD?

1. Lauren Vogel, "Fat Shaming Is Making People Sicker and Heavier," *Canadian Medical Association Journal* 191, no. 23 (2019): E649–49. doi.org /10.1503/cmaj.109-5758.
2. Robertson, Sally, "Obesity is 'not a choice' and fat shaming does not help, says British Psychological Society." News-Medical. www.news-medical .net/news/20190924/Obesity-is-not-a-choice-and-fat-shaming-does-not -help-says-British-Psychological-Society.aspx. (Accessed December 14, 2022.)
3. "count calories," Merriam-Webster.com, accessed August 21, 2022. www .merriam-webster.com/dictionary/countcalories.
4. Elizabeth V. Eikey, "Effects of Diet and Fitness Apps on Eating Disorder Behaviours: Qualitative Study," *BJPsych Open* 7, no. 5 (September 2021): e176. doi.org/10.1192/bjo.2021.1011.

CHAPTER 1

1. Brian Wansink and Jeffrey Sobal, "Mindless Eating: The 200 Daily Food Decisions We Overlook," *Environment and Behavior* 39, no. 1 (January 2007): 106–23. doi.org/10.1177/0013916506295573.

2. Matthew A. Killingsworth and Daniel T. Gilbert, "A Wandering Mind Is an Unhappy Mind," *Science* 330, no. 6006 (Nov 2010): 932. www.science .org/doi/abs/10.1126/science.1192439.

3. "Holiday Weight Gain Is a Worldwide Phenomenon, Study Suggests," Harvard Health Publishing, Harvard Medical School, November 14, 2016. www.health.harvard.edu/diet-and-weight-loss/holiday-weight-gain -is-a-worldwide-phenomenon-study-suggests.

4. Jill Bolte Taylor, *My Stroke of Insight: A Brain Scientist's Personal Journey* (New York: Penguin Books, 2008), 146.

5. P. Rada, N. M. Avena, and B. G. Hoebel, "Daily Bingeing on Sugar Repeatedly Releases Dopamine in the Accumbens Shell," *Neuroscience* 134, no. 3 (2005): 737–44. doi.org/10.1016/j.neuroscience.2005.04.043.

6. David A. Wiss, Nicole Avena, and Pedro Rada, "Sugar Addiction: From Evolution to Revolution," *Front Psychiatry* 9 (November 2018). doi.org/10 .3389/fpsyt.2018.00545.

7. A. Santos-Longhurst, "What Is a Sugar Detox? Effects and How to Avoid Sugar," Healthline.com, August 20, 2020. www.healthline.com/health /sugar-detox-symptoms.

8. Carlo Colantuoni, et al., "Evidence That Intermittent, Excessive Sugar Intake Causes Endogenous Opioid Dependence," *Obesity Research* 10, no. 6 (June 2002): 478–88. doi.org/10.1038/oby.2002.66.

9. Helbert Rondon and Madhu Badireddy, "Hyponatremia," PubMed, Stat-Pearls Publishing, Updated January 2022. www.ncbi.nlm.nih.gov/books /NBK470386/.

CHAPTER 2

1. Lewis Carroll, *Through the Looking-Glass* (United Kingdom: Macmillan, 1871), 39.

2. "Children's Emotional Development Is Built into the Architecture of Their Brains: Working Paper 2," National Scientific Council on the Developing Child (2004), 1. https://developingchild.harvard.edu/resources/childrens -emotional-development-is-built-into-the-architecture-of-their-brains/.

3. Jamie D. Aten, Ph. D., "Wired for Survival. Understand and Harness Your Body's Natural Stress Response when It Counts," *Psychology Today*, June 15, 2017. www.psychologytoday.com/us/blog/heal-and-carry/201706 /wired-survival.

4. Alyson M. Stone, Ph. D., "90 Seconds to Emotional Resilience," Alyson M. Stone, Ph. D., CGP, November 19, 2019. www.alysonmstone.com/90 -seconds-to-emotional-resilience/.

CHAPTER 4

1. "temptation," Oxford Learners Dictionaries, accessed August 21, 2022. www.oxfordlearnersdictionaries.com/us/definition/english/temptation?q =temptation.

2. Wilhelm Hofmann, Roy F. Baumeister, Georg Förster, and Kathleen D. Vohs, "Everyday Temptations: An Experience Sampling Study of Desire, Conflict, and Self-Control," *Journal of Personality and Social Psychology* 102, no. 6 (2012): 1318–35. doi.org/10.1037/a0026545.

3. Marina Milyavskaya, Michael Inzlicht, Nora Hope, and Richard Koestner, "Saying 'No' to Temptation: *Want-to* Motivation Improves Self-Regulation by Reducing Temptation Rather than by Increasing Self-Control," *Journal of Personality and Social Psychology* 109, no. 4 (2015): 677–93. doi.org/10.1037/pspp0000045.

4. Brian M. Galla and Angela L. Duckworth, "More than Resisting Temptation: Beneficial Habits Mediate the Relationship Between Self-Control and Positive Life Outcomes," *Journal of Personality and Social Psychology* 109, no. 3 (2015): 508–25. doi.org/10.1037/pspp0000026.

CHAPTER 5

1. Jie Li, et al., "Improvement in Chewing Activity Reduces Energy Intake in One Meal and Modulates Plasma Gut Hormone Concentrations in Obese and Lean Young Chinese Men," *The American Journal of Clinical Nutrition* 94, no. 3 (September 2011): 709–716. doi.org/10.3945/ajcn.111 .015164.

2. Shah, "Slower Eating Speed Lowers Energy Intake in Normal-Weight but not Overweight/Obese Subjects," 393–402.

3. Matthew Hoffman, "Picture of the Esophagus," WebMD, September 11, 2009. www.webmd.com/digestive-disorders/picture-of-the-esophagus#1.

4. Mark Hsu, Anthony O. Safadi, and Forshing Lui, "Physiology, Stomach." National Library of Medicine, StatPearls Publishing, last updated July 18, 2022. www.ncbi.nlm.nih.gov/books/NBK535425/.

5. Ananya Mandal, "What Does the Small Intestine Do?" News Medical Life Sciences, last updated June 28, 2019. www.news-medical.net/health /What-Does-the-Small-Intestine-Do.aspx.

6. Linda Chia-Hui Yu, "Intestinal Epithelial Barrier Dysfunction in Food Hypersensitivity," *Journal of Allergy* vol. 2012 (2012): 1–11. doi.org/10 .1155/2012/596081.

7. Laura L. Azzouz and Sandeep Sharma, "Physiology, Large Intestine," National Library of Medicine, StatPearls Publishing, last updated August 9, 2021. www.ncbi.nlm.nih.gov/books/NBK507857/.

8. "Primary Functions of the Liver," Health Interactive, 1999. www.rnceus .com/lf/lffx.html.

9. "The Liver & Blood Sugar," Diabetes Education Online, University of California, San Francisco, accessed October 24, 2022. https://dtc.ucsf.edu /types-of-diabetes/type1/understanding-type-1-diabetes/how-the-body -processes-sugar/the-liver-blood-sugar/.

10. J. P. Chaput and A. Tremblay, "The Glucostatic Theory of Appetite Control and the Risk of Obesity and Diabetes," *International Journal of Obesity* 33, no. 1 (2009): 46–53. doi.org/10.1038/ijo.2008.221.

CHAPTER 6

1. Ron Sender, Shai Fuchs, and Ron Milo, "Revised Estimates for the Number of Human and Bacteria Cells in the Body," *PLOS Biology* 14, no. 8 (August 19, 2016): e1002533. doi.org/10.1371/journal.pbio.1002533.

2. Satish S. C. Rao, and Jigat Bhagatwala, "Small Intestinal Bacterial Overgrowth: Clinical Features and Therapeutic Management," *Clinical and Translational Gastroenterology* 10, no. 10 (October 2019): e00078. doi.org /10.14309/ctg.0000000000000078.

3. Askin Erdogan and Satish S. C. Rao, "Small Intestinal Fungal Over-growth," *Current Gastroenterology Reports* 17, no. 4 (April 2015): 16. doi .org/10.1007/s11894-015-0436-2.

4. Elvia Ramírez-Carrillo, et al., "Disturbance in Human Gut Microbiota Networks by Parasites and Its Implications in the Incidence of Depression," *Scientific Reports* 10, no. 1 (2020): 3680. doi.org/10.1038/s41598-020-60562-w.

5. "NIH Human Microbiome Project Defines Normal Bacterial Make Up of the Body," National Institutes of Health, June 13, 2012. www.nih.gov/news -events/news-releases/nih-human-microbiome-project-defines-normal -bacterial-makeup-body#:~:text=The%20human%20body%20contains %20trillions,vital%20role%20in%20human%20health.

6. Wanpen Turakitwanakan, Chantana Mekseepralard, and Panaree Busar-akumtragul, "Effects of Mindfulness Meditation on Serum Cortisol of Medical Students," *Journal of the Medical Association of Thailand* 96, no. 1 (January 2013): 90–5. https://pubmed.ncbi.nlm.nih.gov/23724462/.

CHAPTER 7

1. Killingsworth and Gilbert, "A Wandering Mind is an Unhappy Mind," 932.

2. David T. Neal, Wendy Wood, Mengju Wu, and David Kurlander, "The Pull of the Past: When Do Habits Persist Despite Conflict with Motives?" *Personality and Social Psychology Bulletin* 37, no. 11 (2011): 1428–37. doi.org /10.1177/0146167211419863.

3. Brian Wansink, James E. Painter, and Jill North, "Bottomless Bowls: Why Visual Cues of Portion Size May Influence Intake," *Obesity Research* 13, no. 1 (2005): 93–100. doi.org/10.1038/oby.2005.12.

4. Carolyn M. Pearson, et al., "Investigating the Reinforcing Value of Binge Anticipation," *International Journal of Eating Disorders* 49, no. 6 (2016): 539–41. doi.org/10.1002/eat.22547.

5. Pearson, et al., "Investigating the Reinforcing Value of Binge Anticipation," 539–41.

6. Remez Sasson, "How Many Thoughts Does Your Mind Think in One Hour?" Success Consciousness, accessed October 24, 2022. www.success consciousness.com/blog/inner-peace/how-many-thoughts-does-your -mind-think-in-one-hour/.

CHAPTER 9

1. Samuele M. Marcora, Walter Staiano, and Victoria Manning, "Mental Fatigue Impairs Physical Performance in Humans," *Journal of Applied Physiology* 106, no. 3 (March 2009): 857–64. doi.org/10.1152/japplphysiol .91324.2008.

2. Suzana Herculano-Houzel, "The Human Brain in Numbers: a Linearly Scaled-Up Primate Brain," *Frontiers in Human Neuroscience* 3, no. 31 (2009). doi.org/10.3389/neuro.09.031.2009.

3. Arlin Cunci, "What Happens to Your Body When You're Thinking?" Very-well Mind, Dotdash Meredith, updated July 17, 2019. www.verywellmind .com/what-happens-when-you-think-4688619.

CHAPTER 10

1. Sana Saif, "Weight Loss is 90% Diet and 10% Exercise, Say Experts," *Express Tribune*, November 13, 2017. https://tribune.com.pk/story/1556643 /weight-loss-90-diet-10-exercise-say-experts.

2. C. Tudor-Locke, et al., "How Many Steps/Day Are Enough? For Adults," *International Journal of Behavioral Nutrition and Physical Activity* 3, no. 1 (2011): 79. doi.org/10.1186/1479-5868-8-79.

3. David R. Bassett, Lindsay P. Toth, Samuel R. LaMunion, and Scott E. Crouter, "Step Counting: A Review of Measurement Considerations and Health-Related Applications," *Sports Medicine* 47, no. 7 (2016): 1303–15. doi.org/10.1007/s40279-016-0663-1.

4. Tsung-Lin Chiang, et al., "Is the Goal of 12,000 Steps per Day Suffi-cient for Improving Body Composition and Metabolic Syndrome? The Necessity of Combining Exercise Intensity: a Randomized Controlled Trial," *BMC Public Health* 19, no. 1215 (2019). doi.org/10.1186/s12889 -019-7554-y.

5. Pedro F. Saint-Maurice, et al., "Association of Daily Step Count and Step Intensity with Mortality Among US Adults," *JAMA* 323, no. 2 (2020): 1151–60. doi.org/10.1001/jama.2020.1382.

6. University of Massachusetts Amherst, "Meta-Analysis of 15 Studies Reports New Findings on How Many Daily Walking Steps Needed

for Longevity Benefit: Spoiler Alert: It's Fewer than 10,000, Especially for Older Adults," ScienceDaily, March 3, 2022. www.sciencedaily.com /releases/2022/03/220303112207.htm.

7. James Dorling, et al., "Acute and Chronic Effects of Exercise on Appetite, Energy Intake, and Appetite-Related Hormones: The Modulating Effect of Adiposity, Sex, and Habitual Physical Activity," *Nutrients* 10, no. 9 (2018): 1140. doi.org/10.3390/nu10091140.

8. Dorling, "Acute and Chronic Effects of Exercise on Appetite, Energy Intake, and Appetite-Related Hormones," 1140.

9. Rebecca J. Crochiere, et al., "Is Physical Activity a Risk or Protective Factor for Subsequent Dietary Lapses Among Behavioral Weight Loss Participants?" *Health Psychology* 39, no. 3 (2020): 240–44. doi.org/10.1037 /hea0000839.

CHAPTER 11

1. Jeff Minerd, "BMI 27: The New Normal?" Medpage Today, May 10, 2016. www.medpagetoday.com/primarycare/obesity/57821.

2. Yashushi Ohashi, Ken Sakai, Hiroki Hase, and Nobuhiko Joki, "Dry Weight Targeting: The Art and Science of Conventional Hemodialysis," *Seminars in Dialysis* 31, no. 6 (2018): 551–56. doi.org/10.1111/sdi.12721.

3. Ohashi, "Dry Weight Targeting," 551–56.

4. Julia C. Basso and Wendy A. Suzuki, "The Effects of Acute Exercise on Mood, Cognition, Neurophysiology, and Neurochemical Pathways: A Review," *Brain Plasticity* 2, no. 2 (2017): 127–52. doi.org/10.3233/bpl -160040.

CHAPTER 12

1. "Physical Activity and Your Heart," National Heart, Lung, and Blood Institute, accessed October 24, 2022. www.nhlbi.nih.gov/health/heart /physical-activity/types.

2. Harsh Patel, et al., "Aerobic vs Anaerobic Exercise Training Effects on the Cardiovascular System," *World Journal of Cardiology* 9, no. 2 (2017): 134–38. doi.org/10.4330/wjc.v9.i2.134.

3. Wayne Wescott, ACSM Strength Training Guidelines, *ACSM's Health & Fitness Journal* 13, no. 4 (2009): 14–22. doi.org/10.1249/fit.0b013e3181 aaf460.

4. U.S. Department of Health and Human Services, *Activity Guidelines for Americans*, 2nd ed., Washington, DC: 2018.

5. Thaisa Lemos and Dympna Gallagher, "Current Body Composition Measurement Techniques," *Current Opinion Endocrinology and Diabetes and Obesity* 24, no. 5 (2017): 310–14. doi.org/10.1097/med.00000000000 00360.

CHAPTER 13

1. E. Jéquier and F. Constant, "Water as an Essential Nutrient: the Physiological Basis of Hydration," *European Journal of Clinical Nutrition* 64, no. 2 (2009): 115–23. doi.org/10.1038/ejcn.2009.111.

2. Michael Boschmann, et al., "Water-Induced Thermogenesis," *Journal of Clinical Endocrinology and Metabolism* 88, no. 12 (2003): 6015–19. doi.org /10.1210/jc.2003-030780.

3. Naila A. Shaheen, et al., "Public Knowledge of Dehydration and Fluid Intake Practices: Variation by Participants' Characteristics," *BMC Public Health* 18, no. 1 (2018): 1–8. doi.org/10.1186/s12889-018-6252-5.

4. Joseph Pizzorno, "The Kidney Dysfunction Epidemic, Part 1: Causes," *Integrative Medicine: A Clinician's Journal* 14, no. 6 (Dec 2015): 8–13. www .ncbi.nlm.nih.gov/pmc/articles/PMC4718206/.

5. Simon N. Thornton, "Increased Hydration Can Be Associated with Weight Loss," *Frontiers in Nutrition* 3 (2016). doi.org/10.3389/fnut.2016 .00018.

6. C. Maresh, et al., "Effect of Hydration State on Testosterone and Cortisol Responses to Training-Intensity Exercise in Collegiate Runners," *International Journal of Sports Medicine* 27, no. 10 (October 2006): 765–70. doi.org /10.1055/s-2005-872932.

7. Ana Adan, "Cognitive Performance and Dehydration," *Journal of the American College of Nutrition* 31, no. 2 (April 2012): 71–8. doi.org/10.1080 /07315724.2012.10720011.

8. Kathryn Watson and Stacy Sampson, "What Does It Mean When Dehydration Becomes Long-Term and Serious?" Healthline, July 20, 2018. www.healthline.com/health/chronic-dehydration.

9. Barry M. Popkin, Kristen E. D'Anci, and Irwin H. Rosenberg, "Water, Hydration, and Health," *Nutrition Reviews* 69, no. 8 (2010): 439–58. doi .org/10.1111/j.1753-4887.2010.00304.x.

10. Simon N. Thornton, "Increased Hydration Can Be Associated with Weight Loss," *Frontiers in Nutrition* 3 (2016). doi.org/10.3389/fnut.2016 .00018.

11. Isha Shrimanker and Sandeep Bhattarai, "Electrolytes," PubMed, StatPearls Publishing, updated July 26, 2021. https://pubmed.ncbi.nlm.nih .gov/31082167/.

12. Melissa C. Daniels and Barry M. Popkin, "Impact of Water Intake on Energy Intake and Weight Status: a Systematic Review," *Nutrition Reviews* 68, no. 9 (September 2010): 505–21. doi.org/10.1111/j.1753-4887 .2010.00311.x.

13. Hyo-kyung Ryu, Yong-do Kim, Sung-su Heo, and Sang-cheol Kim, "Effect of Carbonated Water Manufactured by a Soda Carbonator on Etched or Sealed Enamel," *The Korean Journal of Orthodontics* 48, no. 1 (January 2018): 48–56. doi.org/10.4041/kjod.2018.48.1.48.

14. "The Importance of Hydration," Harvard T.H. Chan School of Public Health, updated June 22, 2018. www.hsph.harvard.edu/news/hsph-in-the -news/the-importance-of-hydration/.

15. Shaheen, et al., "Public Knowledge of Dehydration and Fluid Intake Practices: Variation by Participants' Characteristics," 1–8.

16. Jianfen Zhang, et al., "Different Amounts of Water Supplementation Improved Cognitive Performance and Mood Among Young Adults after 12 h Water Restriction in Baoding, China: A Randomized Controlled Trial (RCT)," *International Journal of Environmental Research and Public Health* 17, no. 21 (October 2020): 7792. doi.org/10.3390/ijerph17217792.

17. Fahimeh Haghighatdoost, "Drinking Plain Water is Associated with Decreased Risk of Depression and Anxiety in Adults: Results from a Large Cross-Sectional Study," *World Journal of Psychiatry* 8, no. 3 (September 20, 2018): 88–96. doi.org/10.5498/wjp.v8.i3.88.

CHAPTER 14

1. C. Bode and J. C. Bode, "Alcohol's Role in Gastrointestinal Tract Disorders," *Alcohol Health and Research World* 21, no. 1 (1997): 76–83. https://pubmed.ncbi.nlm.nih.gov/15706765/.

2. Anna-Leena Orsama, et al., "Weight Rhythms: Weight Increases During Weekends and Decreases During Weekdays," *Obesity Facts* 7, no. 1 (2014): 36–47. doi.org/10.1159/000356147.

3. Yogita Rochlani, Naga Venkata Pothineni, Swathi Kovelamudi, and Jawahar L. Mehta, "Metabolic Syndrome: Pathophysiology, Management, and Modulation by Natural Compounds," *Therapeutic Advances in Cardiovascular Disease* 11, no. 8 (August 2017): 215–25. doi.org/10.1177/1753944717711379.

4. Darbaz Adnan, Jonathan Trinh, and Faraz Bishehsari, "Inconsistent Eating Time is Associated with Obesity: a Prospective Study," *EXCLI Journal* (January 14, 2022): 300–6. https://pubmed.ncbi.nlm.nih.gov/35368461/.

5. Julie E. Holesh, Sanah Aslam, and Andrew Martin, "Physiology, Carbohydrates," StatPearls Publishing, updated July 26, 2021. www.ncbi.nlm.nih.gov/books/NBK459280/.

6. David H. Wasserman, "Four Grams of Glucose," *American Journal of Physiology-Endocrinology and Metabolism* 296, no. 1 (January 2009): E11–21. doi.org/10.1152/ajpendo.90563.2008.

7. Holesh, "Physiology, Carbohydrates," www.ncbi.nlm.nih.gov/books/NBK459280/.

8. "The Water in You: Water and the Human Body," USGS, May 22, 2019, U.S. Department of the Interior. www.usgs.gov/special-topic/water-science-school/science/water-you-water-and-human-body?qt-science_center_objects=0#qt-science_center_objects.

CHAPTER 15

1. T. Bear, M. Philipp, S. Hill, T. Mündel. A preliminary study on how hypohydration affects pain perception. Psychophysiology. May 2016; 53 (5): 605-10. doi: 10.1111/psyp.12610. Epub Jan 20, 2016. PMID: 26785699.

2. K. Saketkhoo, A. Januszkiewicz, and M. A. Sackner, "Effects of Drinking Hot Water, Cold Water, and Chicken Soup on Nasal Mucus Velocity and Nasal Airflow Resistance," *CHEST Journal* 74, no. 4 (October 1978): 408–10. doi.org/10.1016/S0012-3692(15)37387-6.

3. Hassan Tariq, et al., "Sips of the Water for the Management of Gastroesophageal Reflux Induced Refractory Cough: a Case Report and Review of the Literature," *Case Reports in Gastrointestinal Medicine* 2019 (June 3, 2019). doi.org/10.1155/2019/9205259.

4. Yu-Rin Kim, "Analysis of the Effect of Daily Water Intake on Oral Health: Result from Seven Waves of a Population-Based Panel Study," *Water* 13, no. 19 (2021): 2716. doi.org/10.3390/w13192716.

CHAPTER 16

1. Goran Medic, Micheline Wille, and Michiel Hemels, "Short- and Long-Term Health Consequences of Sleep Disruption," *Nature and Science of Sleep* 9, no. 9 (May 19, 2017): 151–61. doi.org/10.2147/nss.s134864.

2. Stephanie M. Greer, Andrea N. Goldstein, and Matthew P. Walker, "The Impact of Sleep Deprivation on Food Desire in the Human Brain," *Nature Communications* 4, no. 1 (2013). doi.org/10.1038/ncomms3259.

3. R. R. Markwald, et al., "Impact of insufficient sleep on total daily energy expenditure, food intake, and weight gain," *Proceedings of the National Academy of Sciences* 110, no. 14 (April 2, 2013): 5695-700. https://doi.org/10.1073/pnas.1216951110.

4. Greer, "The Impact of Sleep Deprivation on Food Desire in the Human Brain." doi.org/10.1038/ncomms3259.

5. Vikesh Khanijow, et al., "Sleep Dysfunction and Gastrointestinal Diseases," *Gastroenterol Hepatol (N Y)* 11, no. 12 (December 2015): 817–25. https://pubmed.ncbi.nlm.nih.gov/27134599/.

6. Hung-Ming Chang, "Sleep Deprivation Predisposes Liver to Oxidative Stress and Phospholipid Damage: a Quantitative Molecular Imaging Study," *Journal of Anatomy* 212, no. 3 (March 2008): 295–305. doi.org/10.1111/j.1469-7580.2008.00860.x.

7. Vilma Aho, et al., "Prolonged Sleep Restriction Induces Changes in Pathways Involved in Cholesterol Metabolism and Inflammatory Responses," *Scientific Reports* 6, no. 1 (April 22, 2016). doi.org/10.1038/srep24828.

8. Matthew P. Walker, *Why We Sleep: Unlocking the Power of Sleep and Dreams* (New York: Simon & Schuster, 2017): 134–140.

9. Pleunie S. Hogenkamp, et al., "Acute Sleep Deprivation Increases Portion Size and Affects Food Choice in Young Men," *Psychoneuroendocrinology* 38, no. 9 (September 2013): 1668–74. doi.org/10.1016/j.psyneuen.2013.01 .012.

10. A. V. Nedeltcheva, et al., "Insufficient Sleep, Diet, and Obesity," *Annals of Internal Medicine* 153, no. 7 (October 5, 2010): 435–41. doi.org/10.7326 /0003-4819-153-7-201010050-00002.

11. George P. Chrousos, "Stress and Disorders of the Stress System," *Nature Reviews Endocrinology* 5, no. 7 (July 2009): 374–81. doi.org/10.1038/nrendo .2009.106.

12. Mahita Kadmiel and John A. Cidlowski, "Glucocorticoid Receptor Signaling in Health and Disease," *Trends in Pharmacological Sciences* 34, no. 9 (September 1, 2013): 518–30. www.ncbi.nlm.nih.gov/pmc/articles/PMC 3951203/.

13. Kadmiel, "Glucocorticoid Receptor Signaling in Health and Disease," 518–30.

14. Carol Jones and Christopher Gwenin, "Cortisol Level Dysregulation and Its Prevalence—Is It Nature's Alarm Clock?" *Physiological Reports* 8, no. 24 (January 2021). doi.org/10.14814/phy2.14644.

15. Juan José Hernández Morante, et al., "Moderate Weight Loss Modifies Leptin and Ghrelin Synthesis Rhythms but Not the Subjective Sensations of Appetite in Obesity Patients," *Nutrients* 12, no. 4 (March 27, 2020): 916. doi.org/10.3390/nu12040916.

16. Gwenin, "Cortisol Level Dysregulation and Its Prevalence—Is It Nature's Alarm Clock?" doi.org/10.14814/phy2.14644.

17. "Adrenal Insufficiency (Addison's Disease)," Johns Hopkins Medicine, accessed October 31, 2022. www.hopkinsmedicine.org/health/conditions -and-diseases/underactive-adrenal-glands--addisons-disease.

18. Maria Bantounou, Josip Plascevic, and Helen F. Galley, "Melatonin and Related Compounds: Antioxidant and Anti-Inflammatory Actions," *Antioxidants* 11, no. 3 (2022): 532. doi.org/10.3390/antiox11030532.

19. Russel J. Reiter, et al., "Melatonin as an Antioxidant: Under Promises but Over Delivers," *Journal of Pineal Research* 61, no. 3 (October 2016): 253–78. doi.org/10.1111/jpi.12360.

20. Rüdiger Hardeland, "Neurobiology, Pathophysiology, and Treatment of Melatonin Deficiency and Dysfunction," *The Scientific World Journal* 2012: 1–18. doi.org/10.1100/2012/640389.

21. Lauren A. E. Erland and Praveen K. Saxena, "Melatonin Natural Health Products and Supplements: Presence of Serotonin and Significant Variability of Melatonin Content," *Journal of Clinical Sleep Medicine* 13, no. 2 (2017): 275–81. https://pubmed.ncbi.nlm.nih.gov/27855744/.

22. Michael J. Sateia, et al., "Clinical Practice Guideline for the Pharmacologic Treatment of Chronic Insomnia in Adults: an American Academy of Sleep Medicine Clinical Practice Guideline," *Journal of Clinical Sleep Medicine* 13, no. 2 (2017): 307–49. doi.org/10.5664/jcsm.6470.

23. Jericho Hallare and Valerie Gerriets, "Half Life," National Library of Medicine, StatPearls Publishing, updated June 22, 2022. https://www.ncbi.nlm.nih.gov/books/NBK554498/.

24. C. E. Koch, et al., "Interaction between Circadian Rhythms and Stress," *Neurobiological Stress* 6 (September 8, 2017): 57–67. https://pubmed.ncbi.nlm.nih.gov/28229109/.

25. Sanjay R. Patel, et al., "Association Between Reduced Sleep and Weight Gain in Women," *American Journal of Epidemiology* 164, no. 10 (November 15, 2006): 946–54. doi.org/10.1093/aje/kwj280.

26. Kelly M. Ness, et al., "Four Nights of Sleep Restriction Suppress the Postprandial Lipemic Response and Decrease Satiety," *Journal of Lipid Research* 60, no. 11 (November 2019): 1935–45. doi.org/10.1194/jlr.P094375.

27. Hans K. Meier-Ewert, "Effect of Sleep Loss on C-Reactive Protein, an Inflammatory Marker of Cardiovascular Risk," *Journal of the American College of Cardiology* 43, no. 4 (February 18, 2004): 678–83. doi.org/10.1016/j.jacc.2003.07.050.

28. Koloud Althakafi, et al., "Prevalence of short sleep duration and effect of co-morbid medical conditions—A cross-sectional study in Saudi Arabia," *Journal of Family Medicine and Primary Care* 8, no. 10 (October 31, 2019): 3334-39. doi.org/10.4103/jfmpc.jfmpc_660_19.

29. Christopher M. Depner, et al., "Ad Libitum Weekend Recovery Sleep Fails to Prevent Metabolic Dysregulation During a Repeating Pattern of Insufficient Sleep and Weekend Recovery Sleep," *Current Biology* 29, no. 6 (March 18, 2019): 957–67. doi.org/10.1016/j.cub.2019.01.069.

30. Shingo Kitamura, et al., "Estimating Individual Optimal Sleep Duration and Potential Sleep Debt," *Scientific Reports* 6, no. 1 (2016). doi.org/10.1038/srep35812.

31. Max Hirshkowitz, et al., "The National Sleep Foundation's Sleep Time Duration Recommendations: Methodology and Results Summary," *Sleep Health* 1, no. 1 (2015): 40–3.

32. Nathaniel F. Watson, et al., "Recommended Amount of Sleep for a Healthy Adult: a Joint Consensus Statement of the American Academy of Sleep Medicine and Sleep Research Society," *Sleep* 38, no. 6 (June 2015): 843–4. doi.org/10.5665/sleep.4716.

33. Althakafi, et al., "Prevalence of Short Sleep Duration and Effect of Co-Morbid Medical Conditions," 3334–39.

34. Jean-Phillippe Chaput, Jean-Pierre Després, Claude Bouchard, and Angelo Tremblay, "The Association Between Sleep Duration and Weight Gain in Adults: a 6-Year Prospective Study from the Quebec Family Study," *Sleep* 31, no. 4 (April 2008): 517–23. doi.org/10.1093/sleep/31.4.517.

35. Michael J. Wheeler, et al., "Distinct Effects of Acute Exercise and Breaks in Sitting on Working Memory and Executive Function in Older Adults: a Three-Arm, Randomised Cross-Over Trial to Evaluate the Effects of Exercise with and Without Breaks in Sitting on Cognition," *British Journal of Sports Medicine* (2019). doi.org/10.1136/bjsports-2018-100168.

CHAPTER 17

1. Cassie J. Hilditch, Jillian Dorrian, and Siobhan Banks, "Time to Wake Up: Reactive Countermeasures to Sleep Inertia," *Industrial Health* 54, no. 6 (December 7, 2016): 528–41. doi.org/10.2486/indhealth.2015-0236.

2. Amber Brooks and Leon Lack, "A Brief Afternoon Nap Following Nocturnal Sleep Restriction: Which Nap Duration is Most Recuperative?" *Sleep* 29, no. 6 (June 2006): 831–40. doi.org/10.1093/sleep/29.6.831.

3. V. C. Abad and C. Guilleminault, "Diagnosis and Treatment of Sleep Disorders: a Brief Review for Clinicians," *Chronobiology and Mood Disorders* 5, no. 4 (December 2003): 371–88. doi.org/10.31887/dcns.2003.5.4/vabad.

4. Abad, "Diagnosis and Treatment of Sleep Disorders: a Brief Review for Clinicians," 371–88.

5. Sonia Ancoli-Israel, Donald L. Bliwise, and Jens Peter Nørgaard, "The Effect of Nocturia on Sleep," *Sleep Medicine Reviews* 15, no. 2 (April 2011): 91–7. doi.org/10.1016/j.smrv.2010.03.002.

6. Centers for Disease Control and Prevention, "Perceived Insufficient Rest or Sleep Among Adults—United States," *Morbidity and Mortality Weekly Report* 58, no. 42 (October 31, 2009): 1175–79. www.cdc.gov/mmwr/preview/mmwrhtml/mm5842a2.htm.

7. Mahesh M. Thakkar, Rishi Sharma, and Predeep Sahota, "Alcohol Disrupts Sleep Homeostasis," *Alcohol* 49, no. 4 (2015). doi.org/10.1016/j.alcohol.2014.07.019.

8. M. Basner, C. Clark, A. Hansell, J. I. Hileman, S. Janssen, K. Shepherd, V. Sparrow. Aviation Noise Impacts: State of the Science. Noise Health. 2017 Mar-Apr; 19 (87): 41-50. doi: 10.4103/nah.NAH_104_16. PMID: 29192612; PMCID: PMC5437751.

9. M. M. Ohayon, C. Milesi. Artificial Outdoor Nighttime Lights Associate with Altered Sleep Behavior in the American General Population. Sleep. 2016 Jun 1; 39 (6): 1311-20. doi: 10.5665/sleep.5860. PMID: 27091523; PMCID: PMC4863221.

CHAPTER 18

1. Megan E. Jewett, et al., "Time Course of Sleep Inertia Dissipation in Human Performance and Alertness," *Journal of Sleep Research* 8, no. 1 (October 2008): 1–8. doi.org/10.1111/j.1365-2869.1999.00128.x.

2. M. Nathaniel Mead, "Benefits of Sunlight: a Bright Spot for Human Health," *Environmental Health Perspectives* 116, no. 4 (April 2008): 160–7. doi.org/10.1289/ehp.116-a160.

3. Shia T. Kent, et al., "Effect of Sunlight Exposure on Cognitive Function Among Depressed and Non-Depressed Participants: a REGARDS Cross-Sectional Study," *Environmental Health* 8, no. 1 (July 28, 2009). doi .org/10.1186/1476-069x-8-34.

4. Thaneeya Hawiset, "Effect of One-Time Coffee Fragrance Inhalation on Working Memory, Mood, and Salivary Cortisol Level in Healthy Young Volunteers: a Randomized Placebo Controlled Trial," *Integrative Medicine Research* 8, no. 4 (December 2019): 273–78. doi.org/10.1016/j.imr.2019 .11.007.

5. Ana Kovacevic, Barbara Fenesi, Emily Paolucci, and Jennifer J. Heisz, "The Effects of Aerobic Exercise Intensity on Memory in Older Adults," *Applied Physiology, Nutrition, and Metabolism* (October 2019): 591–600. doi.org/10.1139/apnm-2019-0495.

6. Paul Montgomery and Jane Dennis, "A Systematic Review of Non-Pharmacological Therapies for Problems in Later Life," *Sleep Medicine Reviews* 8, no. 1 (2004): 47–62. doi.org/10.1016/s1087-0792(03)00 026-1.

7. Su I Iao, et al., "Associations Between Bedtime Eating or Drinking, Sleep Duration and Wake After Sleep Onset: Findings from the American Time Use Survey," *British Journal of Nutrition* (September 2021): 1888–97. doi.org/10.1017/s0007114521003597.

8. Iao, "Associations Between Bedtime Eating or Drinking, Sleep Duration and Wake After Sleep Onset," 1888–97.

9. Amber Kinsey and Michael Ormsbee, "The Health Impact of Nighttime Eating: Old and New Perspectives," *Nutrients* 7, no. 4 (April 9, 2015): 2648–62. doi.org/10.3390/nu7042648.

10. Ian M. Colrain, Christian L. Nicholas, and Fiona C. Baker, "Alcohol and the Sleeping Brain," *Handbook of Clinical Neurology* (2014): 415–31. doi.org /10.1016/b978-0-444-62619-6.00024-0.

11. Timothy Roehrs, Kate Papineau, Leon Rosenthal, and Thomas Roth, "Ethanol as a Hypnotic in Insomniacs: Self Administration and Effects

on Sleep and Mood," *Neuropsychopharmacology* 20, no. 3 (1999): 279–86. doi.org/10.1016/S0893-133X(98)00068-2.

12. Roehrs, "Ethanol as a Hypnotic in Insomniacs," 279–86.

13. Joshua J. Gooley, et al., "Exposure to Room Light Before Bedtime Suppresses Melatonin Onset and Shortens Melatonin Duration in Humans," *Journal of Clinical Endocrinology and Metabolism* 96, no. 3 (March 2011): E463–72. doi.org/10.1210/jc.2010-2098.

ABOUT THE AUTHOR

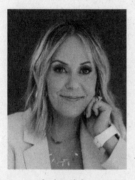 **Kim Shapira** is a Registered Dietitian. She received her BS from Tulane University and her MS from Boston University with an emphasis in Human Metabolism and Clinical Nutrition. She has been in private practice for over two decades, taught nutrition at California State University, Northridge (CSUN), and created the Kim Shapira Method. In her work with her clients, she realized that, while losing weight is very important in one's health journey, having a healthy relationship with food was the most important component in keeping the weight off and finding sustainable health. Kim uses her method daily with clients privately and in group sessions. Kim lives in Los Angeles with her husband, three daughters, and three fur babies. *This Is What You're Really Hungry For* is her first book.

kimshapiramethod.com
@kimshapiramethod

For more ways to implement the
six simple rules into your life,
follow Kim on all social media platforms
@kimshapiramethod.

In addition, Kim offers one-on-one
sessions, virtual group therapy sessions,
and virtual classes on mastering the
six simple rules. Plus there's a weekly
newsletter and blog full of tips and tricks.